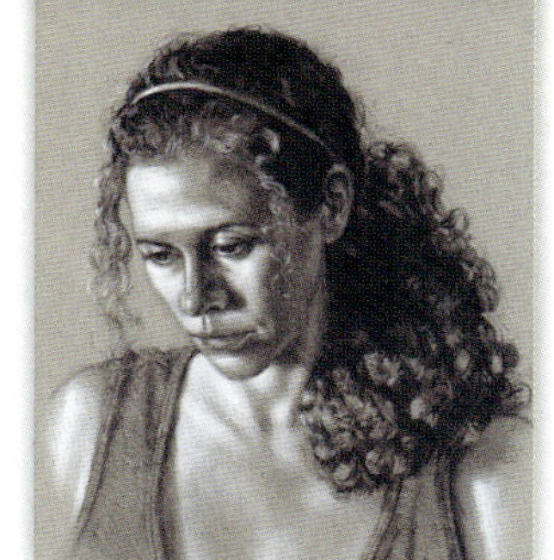

# The Head

**Understanding and replicating** the human figure as portraiture is a classical art form from ancient Greece. Subjects throughout history have utilized the art of the portrait to have their character and likeness immortalized for future generations to see.

You'll find that learning to draw the human head is a challenging but rewarding experience. To guide you along your way, this book contains the basic elements, principles, and approaches involved in the construction of a portrait. You will follow along with step-by-step projects and study topics gathered from my experience in the studio, on the street, and while teaching in the classroom. Winning my first art contest when I was five years old instilled a relentless passion and fire in my soul for drawing and portraiture. This book is helpful for both beginners and the advanced student. Talent is easy to find in this world; however, the level of success you reach and the draftsmanship skills you obtain will come from drawing from life, hard work, study, and practice. Capturing a likeness and creating a beautiful portrait is gratifying for both the artist and the subject. When you develop the habit of drawing on a regular basis, you too can realize the art of the portrait and participate in this timeless tradition.

—*Nathan Rohlander*

## CONTENTS



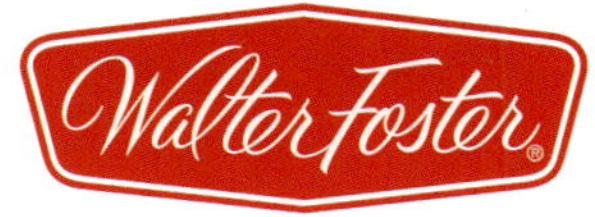

# Materials

The most common drawing medium in this book is graphite, but keep in mind that exploring and experimenting with different drawing mediums will encourage you to create new and fresh drawings. Having a command over a variety of tools facilitates various means of expression.

Being prepared with your tools sharpened and easy to reach will empower you to focus on drawing while the model is on the stand. Models pose for a set number of minutes, so you must be ready to seize the moment!

◀ **Graphite** *Graphite pencils, which contain a mixture of graphite and clay binder, come in a variety of hardnesses. The codes on the pencils are as follows: H stands for the relative hardness of the graphite; the higher the number before the H, the lighter or grayer the mark. B stands for the relative blackness of the pencil and is a softer lead; the higher the number before the B, the blacker the mark. The pencils with F or HB lie in the middle of the value spectrum. Most pencils have a wood exterior containing the graphite core. Another option, and one of my favorites, is the solid graphite pencil or woodless graphite pencil. This tool allows for a wider size range of mark making.*

◀ **Derwent Drawing Pencils** *Creamy earth tone pencils, such as Derwent Drawing Pencils or Conté crayon pencils, come in a range of hues that are great for head drawing. Formulated with a wax binder, the tool glides across the drawing surface like a crayon but can be as precise as graphite.*

◀ **Pastel** *Pastel is a dry, chalky pigment that is useful for drawings with color. A pastel pencil is hard pastel inside a wooden casing. This tool is cleaner than a traditional stick of pastel. Note that hard pastels have more binder than the more buttery soft pastel.*

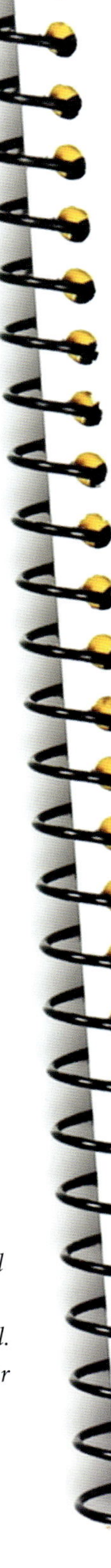

▶ **Chamois** *The artist's chamois is a piece of soft, porous leather or imitation leather. It is used for blending, toning, and gradating charcoal and pastel.*

▶ **Charcoal** *Charcoal can create beautiful, matte black values. This medium comes in both stick and pencil form. Like graphite, charcoal comes in a variety of hardnesses (labeled B for soft and H for hard). Vine and willow charcoal (which come in stick form) create a more sensitive mark than pencils. These forms of charcoal are more temporal and require a fixative or layers of harder charcoal over them to permanently adhere to the paper. They are great for creating even tone on the paper. White charcoal, available in stick and pencil form, is used on toned paper to enhance areas of light. It does not come in a range of hardnesses.*

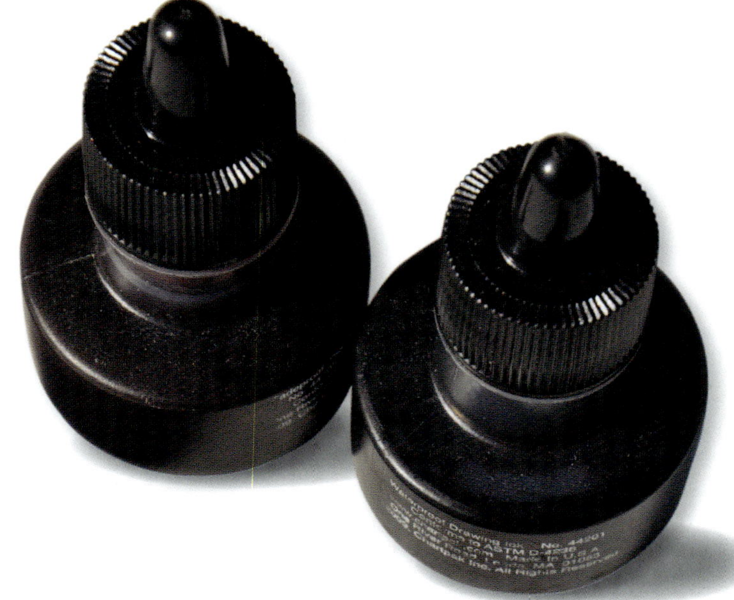

▲ **Drawing Ink** *Although we won't be using ink for the step-by-step projects in this book, it is a common medium in classical drawing. Ink is available in a range of colors, but I most often use black or brown. Black ink straight from the jar can be truly opaque when applied in a few layers. To create transparent washes, mix the ink with water in a separate jar or on a watercolor palette. The ink-to-water ratio determines the level of transparency. I prefer ink containers with an eyedropper cap so I can easily control the amount of ink I add to mixes. I work with waterproof ink; when dry, it does not reactivate beneath subsequent layers.*

▶ **Calligraphy Brush** *This Chinese brush has tapered bristles that are ideal for working with ink. However, you can use any animal-hair or synthetic brush designed for watercolors.*

▲ **Toned Paper** *Toned paper comes in a variety of colors and grays, and you can usually purchase it by the sheet. For head drawing purposes, the most common tones are middle-value neutrals, such as grays and earth tones. These papers are often used with black and white charcoal or pastel. Some papers have a rough and smooth side. I prefer the smooth side, which allows me to render with an even tone. However, the rough side is great for adhering heavy amounts of dry medium to the paper, such as thick applications of pastel or charcoal.*

**Hot-Press Watercolor Paper** *For many of the drawings in this book, I used high quality, hot-press watercolor paper. The paper is archival, which means that it will not yellow or deteriorate with time. Hot press means that the paper is smooth, as though it was pressed with a hot iron. Cold-press papers have more "tooth," or texture. Watercolor paper is a heavy weight and is great for working with wet media.*

**Acetate or Dura-Lar** *Acetate or Dura-Lar drawing surfaces are archival because they are plastic. The plastic, which is frosted and not completely transparent, comes in a matte finish that has an ideal coating for working with both dry and wet media. Both come in a variety of thicknesses. I enjoy working with these because of the smooth, toothless surface and the crisp quality of mark I can achieve.*

▶ **Erasers** *The kneaded eraser is the most versatile eraser on the market. It is a self-cleaning, malleable eraser that can perform a variety of techniques. The kneaded eraser works well with graphite, charcoal, and wax crayon. Another option is a battery-powered eraser, which can recover the white of the paper rapidly whether your medium is charcoal, graphite, or wax. The eraser head allows for great detail.*

▶ **Black Ballpoint Pen** *A black ballpoint pen is an excellent drawing tool. It allows for variation in line weight and forces you to commit to your lines, as you can't erase them. I use this tool for drawing on-the-go in my sketchbook.*

▼ **Metal Divider** *This metal divider can spread open or closed to hold a unit of measurement. You can measure anything you are drawing with this tool, such as the width of an eye. It can also help you determine the length of a facial feature as it relates to another. Lock your elbow as you hold the tool out from your body to avoid fluctuating your unit of measurement.*

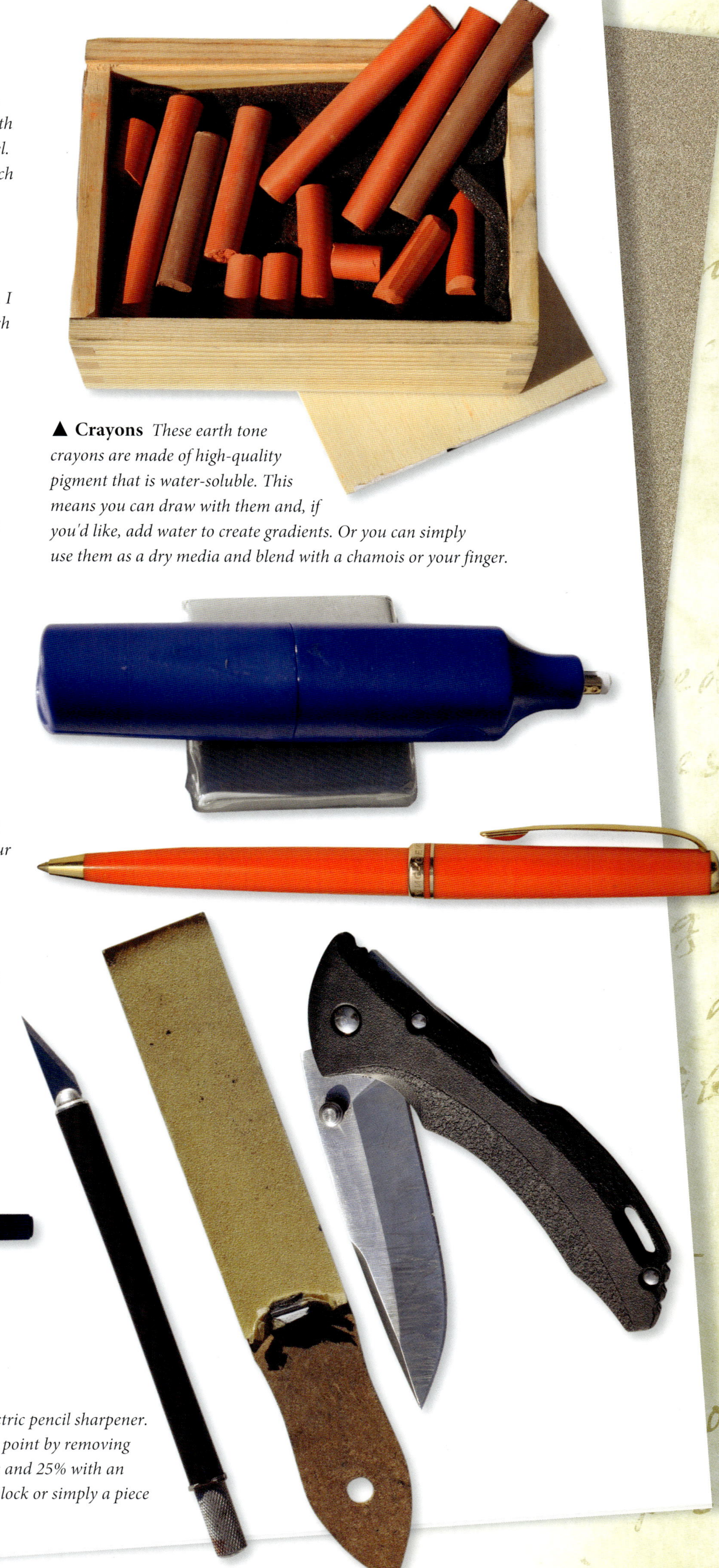

▲ **Crayons** *These earth tone crayons are made of high-quality pigment that is water-soluble. This means you can draw with them and, if you'd like, add water to create gradients. Or you can simply use them as a dry media and blend with a chamois or your finger.*

▶ **Sharpeners** *To sharpen pencils, you can use a utility knife or an electric pencil sharpener. With hand-held blades like a utility knife, you can carve the pencil into a point by removing the wood of the pencil in chunks. I sharpen 75% of my pencils with blades and 25% with an electric sharpener. You can also refine the tip by using an artist sanding block or simply a piece of sandpaper.*

# Measurements and Proportion

**Using a standard set** of measurements helps the artist create accurate proportions when constructing a head drawing. In this section, you'll find measurements that can serve as general guidelines for your head drawings. These proportions are created from averages of the human population at large; however, remember that all people are not the same—they are individuals with varying proportions, and it is these variations that make us different from one another. Solely relying on standard measurements will result in a stylized portrait.

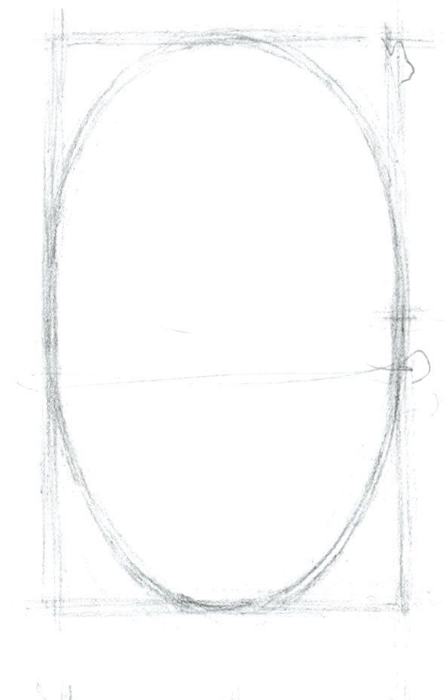

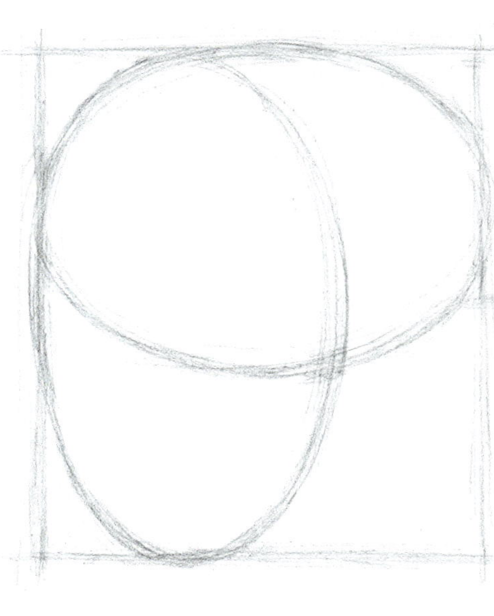

**1.** *Begin with simple shapes first. A) Frontal: Start with a vertical rectangle. Inside, draw a single oval that includes the cranial and facial mass. B) Profile: Begin with a square. Then use two separate ovals connected at the forehead to draw the facial and cranial mass. In both drawings, the halfway point is lightly marked along the vertical line.*

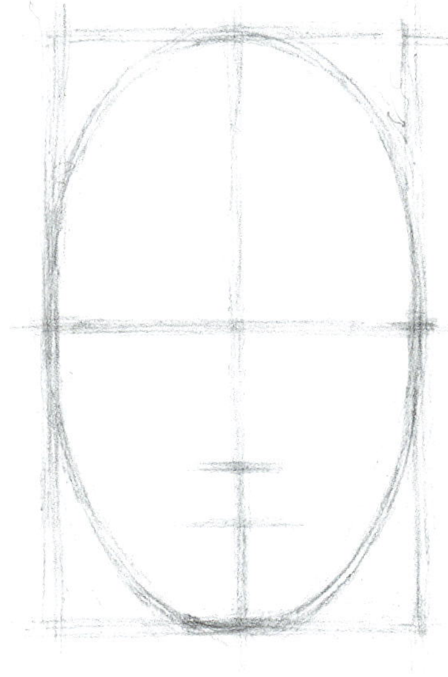

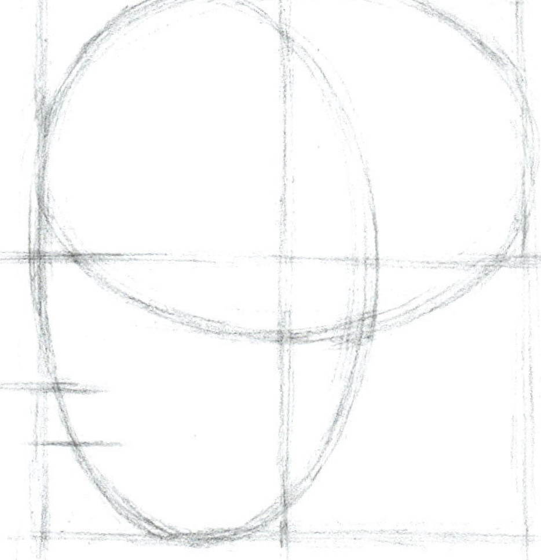

**2.** *A) Frontal: Draw the major axis (vertical) to indicate the centerline of the face. Then add the minor axis (horizontal) to place the eyes. The tops of the eyelids are approximately halfway down the face. Draw a line halfway from the eye line to the chin to mark the base of the nose. The mouth is usually one-third of the way from the base of the nose to the chin. B) Profile: Divide the square into four by drawing a cross in its center. Mark nose and mouth measurements as in the frontal view (A).*

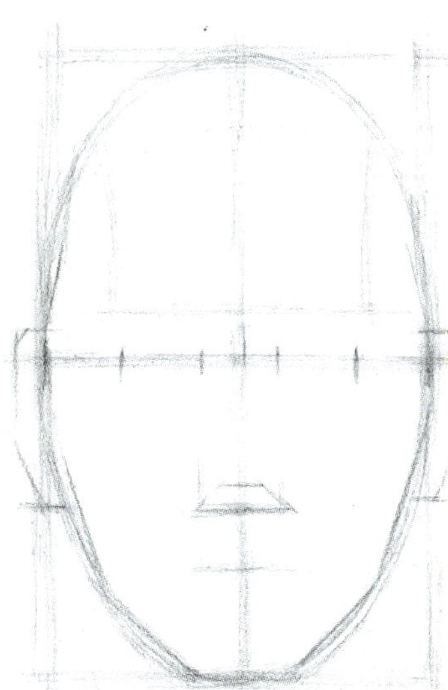

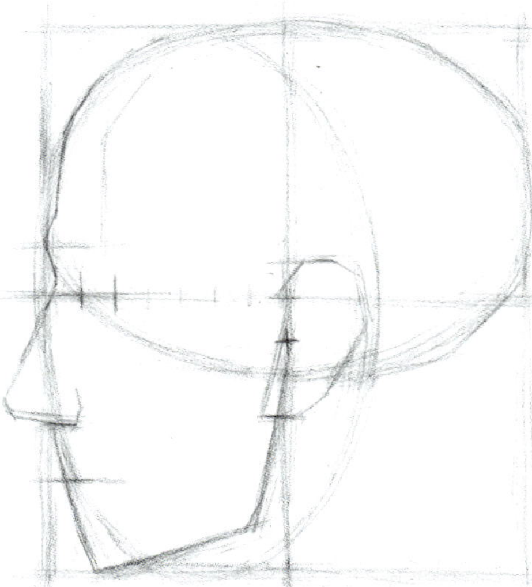

**3.** *A) Frontal: A head is roughly five eyes wide. Divide the eye line into five equal units, with one unit of measurement in the center, between the actual location of the eyes. The tops of the ears are slightly higher than the eye line. The bases of the ears correspond to the base of the nose. Draw the ears with simple shapes first using straight-line segments. Starting with the line for the brow ridge above the eye line, block in the forehead and base of the nose.*

*B) Profile: Indicate the center of the ear in profile with a dark cross slightly below the center of the square. The space from the front of the face to the ear is approximately seven profile eye widths. Other ear measurements correlate with the frontal view. Place the eye approximately two eyes in from the front arch of the face. Now draw the angles of the nose and jawbone. Separate the forehead from the side of the head.*

**4.** *Everything on the face has a front, top, and bottom. When drawing the eyes, start with the eye socket first, using straight lines to create the overall shape. Then move to the upper lid. Articulate the nose with a bridge, sides, and base; then draw the planes of the face. Add the philtrum, which connects the base of the nose to the upper lip. Chisel out the cranial mass further. Develop the ear shapes, making them more organic and specific. Increase the line weight and override the measurement lines.*

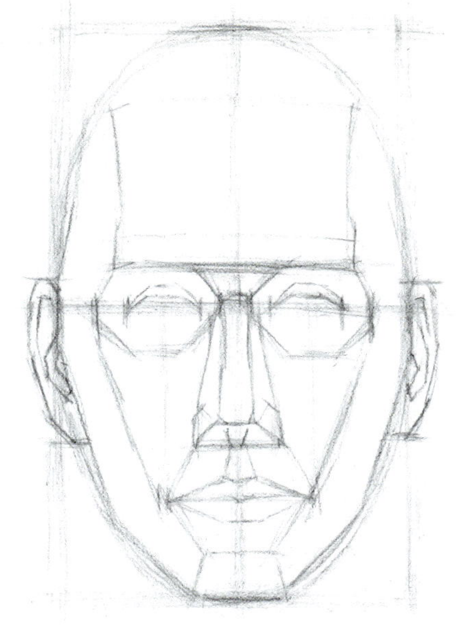

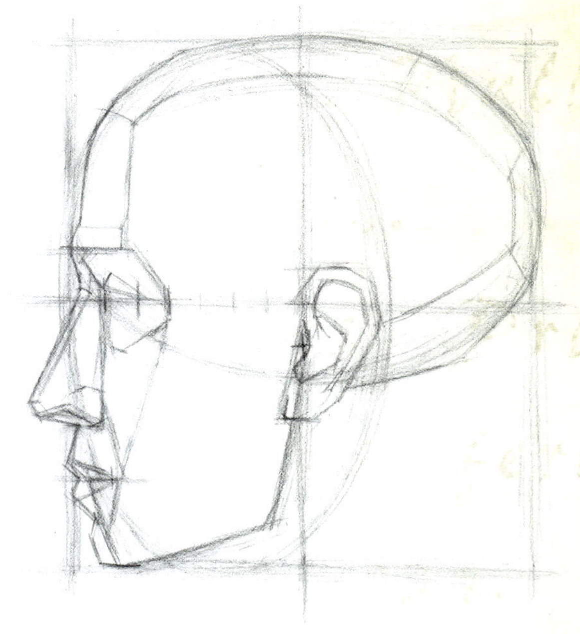

**5.** *Now fluctuate the contour line to reveal the organic qualities of the face. Add the iris and pupil. The upper and lower lids of the eye eclipse portions of the iris. Articulate the eyebrows with simple shapes, and place the nostrils at the base of the nose. Reveal the protuberance of the mouth using lines from the nostrils to the corners of the mouth. Then add the contours of the neck and the hairline to separate the face from the rest of the head.*

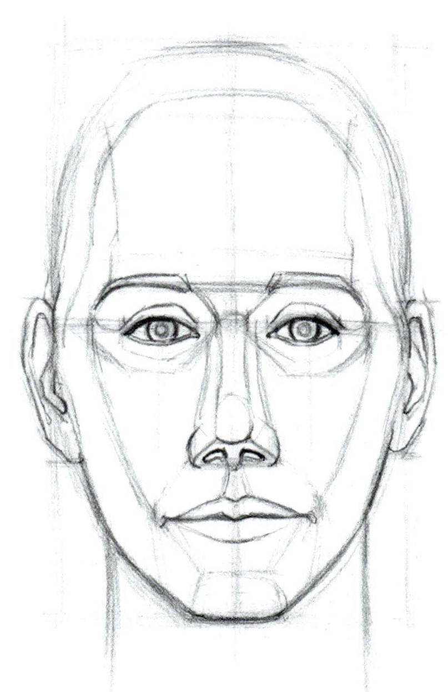

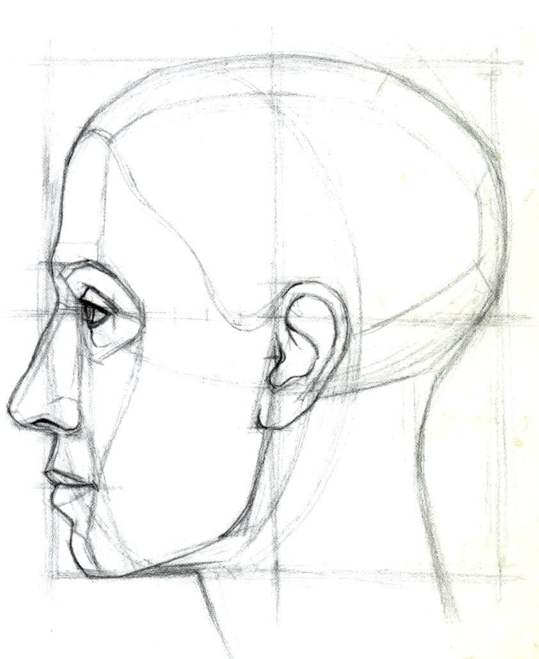

## Measuring and Point of View

***Measuring Your Subject***

**1. From your point of view, hold the divider in your hand, stretch out your arm, and lock your elbow. It is imperative that you keep the divider the same distance between you and what is being measured. Do this every time you check a measurement in a drawing. 2. Spread open the divider and adjust it so that one point is on the top of an eye and the other point is on the base of the chin. You might want to close one eye. This will give you the size of half of the head from your point of view. Use this size as your unit of measurement. 3. You can also measure the figure you're drawing by eye widths. You can see in the diagrams above that the standard face is five eyes wide. Once you've established these measurements, switch to a new unit of measurement, such as the base of the nose to the bottom of the chin. The more you measure and compare, the more accurate your drawings will be!**

***Point of View***

**Always maintain and return to the same point of view when drawing. To help, you can mark your location on the ground with tape. Remember to return your head to the same position or point of view when assessing your work. Even the slightest movement from your original position is problematic. The smallest tilt or change in your head position will change the look of your subject, affecting the relationships of the parts of the figure to the whole. Using your divider will work only if you maintain the same point of view.**

# Meaurements: Foreshortened

**Foreshortening occurs when** parts of an object nearest the viewer appear larger than parts that are farther away. For example, have someone stand in front of you with arms at his or her side. Take note of the size relationship of the hand and the head. Now have the person hold out a hand toward you, palm facing you. Notice that the hand now appears much larger in proportion to the head. This illusion is foreshortening in action.

Applying the rules of perspective and foreshortening help create the illusion of volume and space. Mastering these principles results in more dynamic poses and compositions. Poses and perspectives that involve foreshortening can be more challenging than others. The obstacle is to overcome drawing *what you think you know* and instead draw *what you observe and truly see*. In a three-quarter view of the head, such as the drawings below, the model is looking off to one side. Plenty of beginners make the far side of the face too large and fail to eclipse the tear duct with the bridge of the nose. This is because people are accustomed to seeing a face in frontal view. These beginners are drawing what they think they know—not what is in front of them.

**1.** *Starting with a simple box for the head allows you to see the major planes, indicate whether the model is looking up or down, and establish which side of the head we see. First, lightly draw a rectangle or square—whichever shape best fits your model's head. If the model is looking down and to the right, you should see the top, left side, and front of the box. If the model is looking up and to the left, you should see the bottom, right side, and front of the box.*

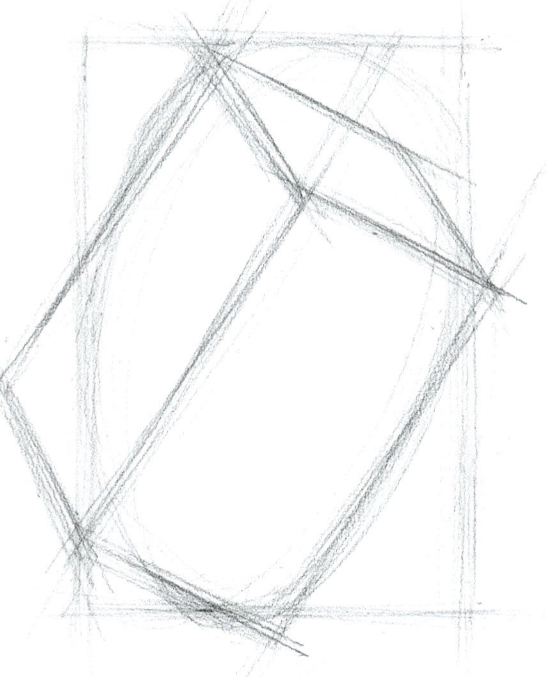

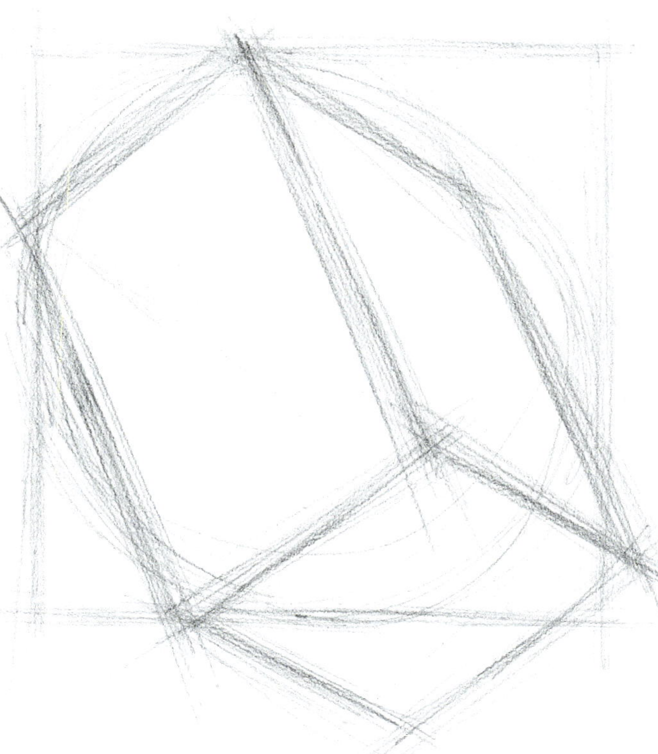

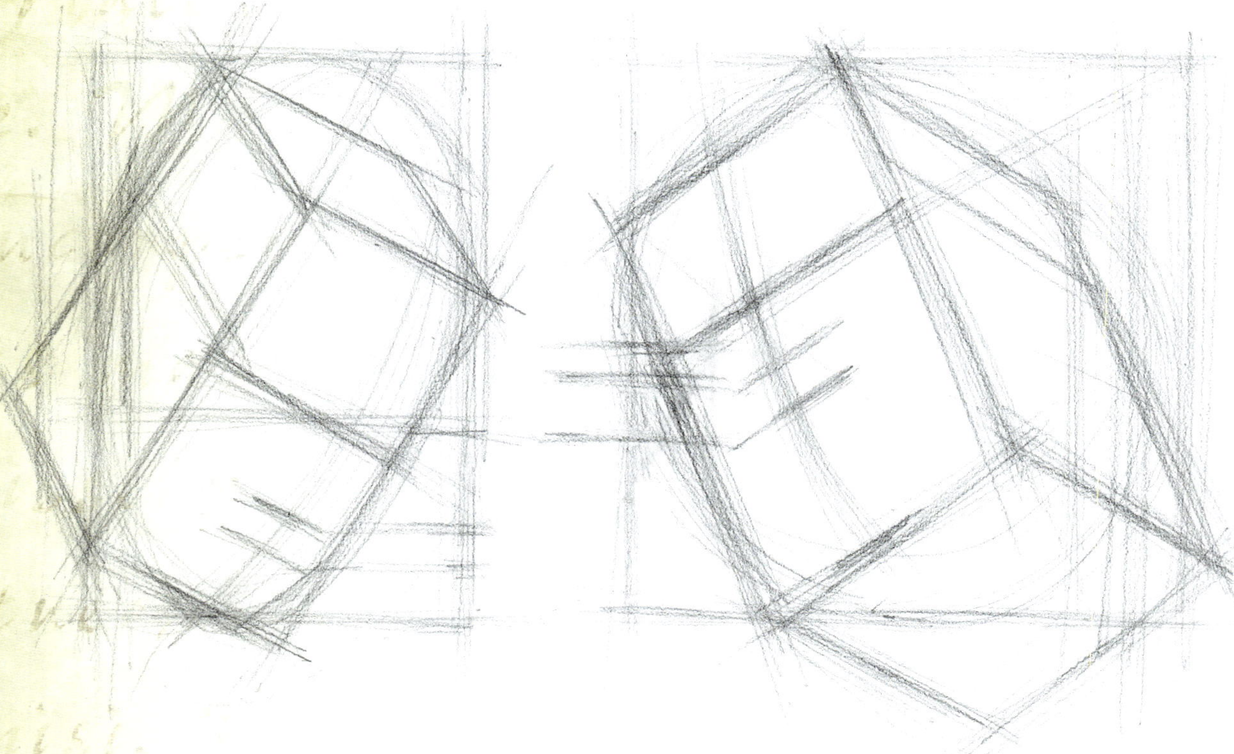

**2.** *Mark the positions of the eyes, nose, mouth, and ears. Notice how foreshortening changes the marks from the frontal and profile views. When the model is looking down, it is important to know where the forehead becomes the top of the head. Then your measurements are easier to place on the front of the face. When the model is looking up, foreshortening appears more extreme. The eyes are high on the front of the face, reducing the amount of forehead seen. Foreshortening changes the ear line in relation to the other measurements and reduces the distances between the eyes, nose, and mouth. Check your angles and measurements—the relationships among features can be deceiving.*

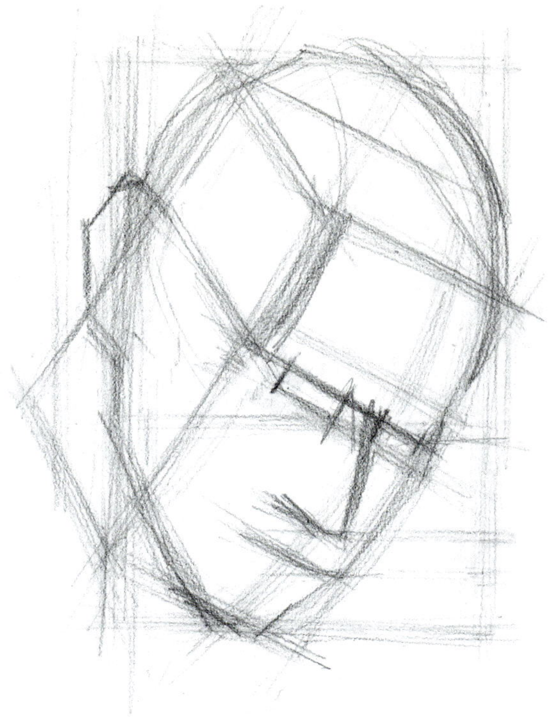

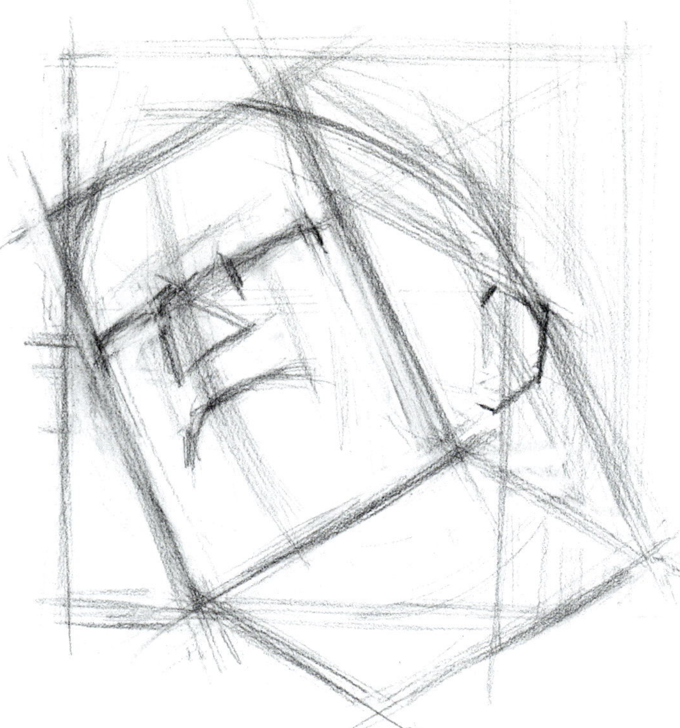

**3.** *Begin chiseling out the shape of the head from the box using straight-line segments. When the model is looking down, we do not see the base of the nose. But when the model is looking up, we see plenty of the base. The arc of the mouth wraps with the curvature of the face and depends on the position of the head. Begin drawing the ears using straight lines that show where the curves change direction. Block in the eyes using rectangles.*

**4.** *Further develop the planes of the head. Build the eye sockets before refining the eyes; this allows you to analyze the shapes around the eye for proper construction. Determine the shapes contained in the ears. When the model is looking down, focus on the bridge of the nose; when the model is looking up, focus on the nostrils. At this point, some straight-line segments should slowly become more organic.*

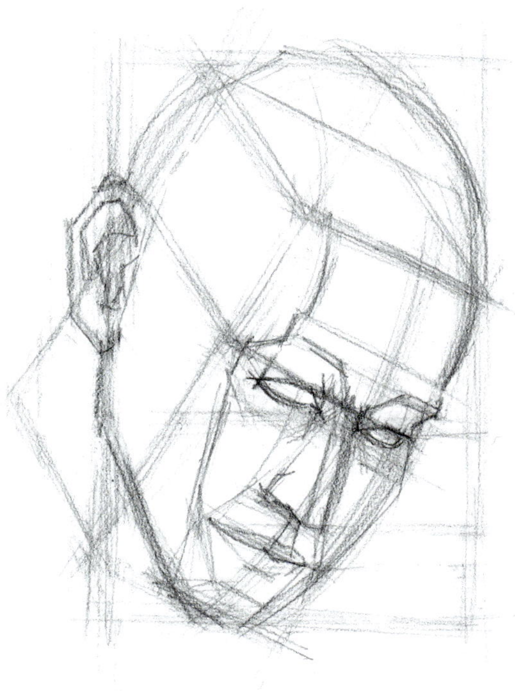

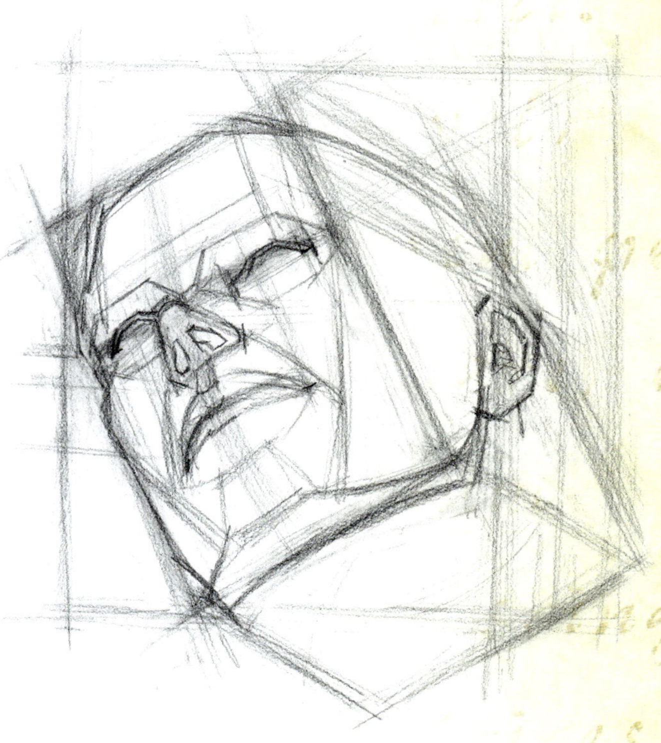

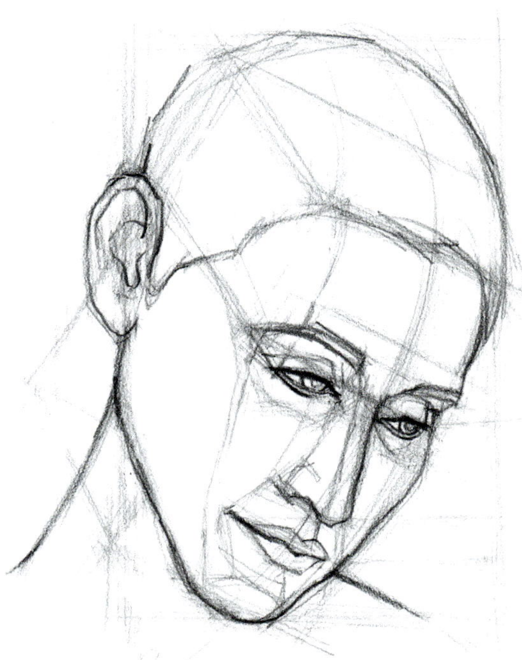

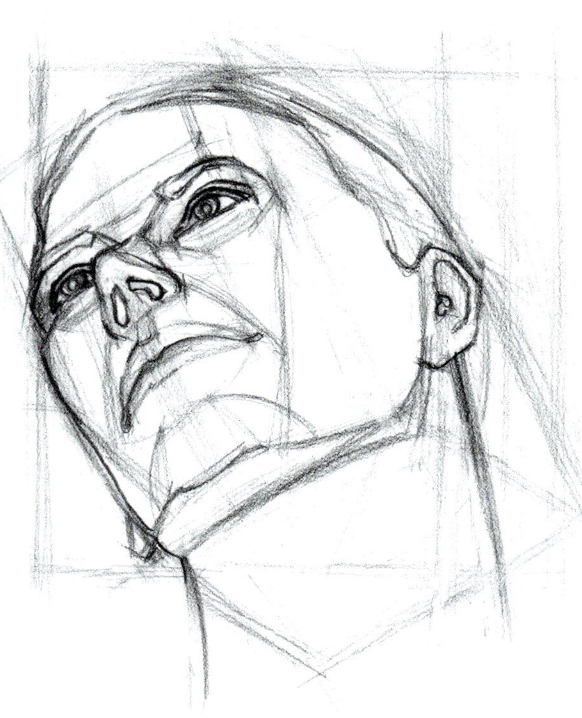

**5.** *In this step, increase your line weight to suggest value and create focal points or areas of interest, such as the eyes. Use more defined contour lines to articulate the organic qualities of the human head and define the major forms. (For more on contour lines, see page 12.) Separate the hair shapes from the "mask" of the face, and add the eyebrows. Draw the contours of the neck as they relate to the gesture of the head.*

# Eyes and Noses

Eyes and noses are important facial features to consider when creating a likeness, and it's necessary to note how closely they relate to each other. Imagine that you are constructing these elements together as one unit. Also, pay attention to any distinguishing features your subject might have. These unique elements require special attention and can make or break your work.

## Eyes

Many artists go straight for the eyes when developing a portrait. I do not recommend this for the beginner. Becoming enraptured by the windows to the soul might compromise your portrait. Simple shapes should be drawn first, and details should be added last. Establishing the shapes of the head that surround the eyes will help with proper placement and proportion within the big picture. It's easier to solve a puzzle if you first place the outside pieces and work your way toward the center.

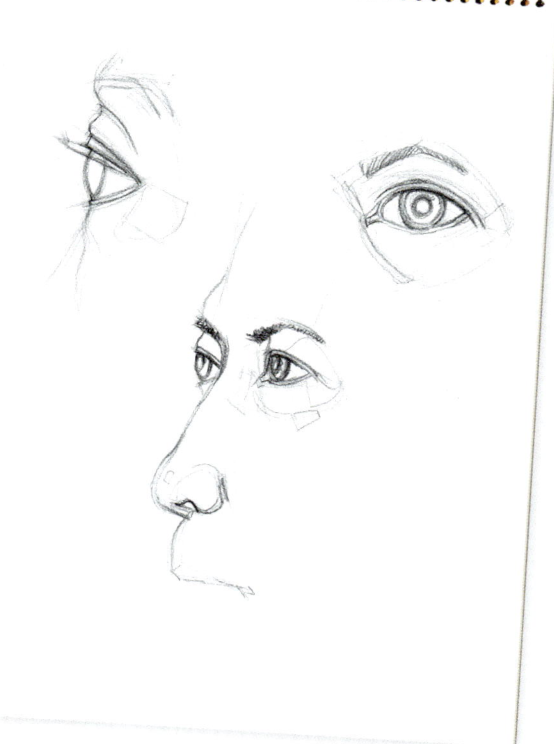

▶ **Eye Study** *Before beginning a final portrait, it's a good idea to study your subject's features and create some quick sketches. This will help you better understand your subject, such as how the eyes and nose relate and connect.*

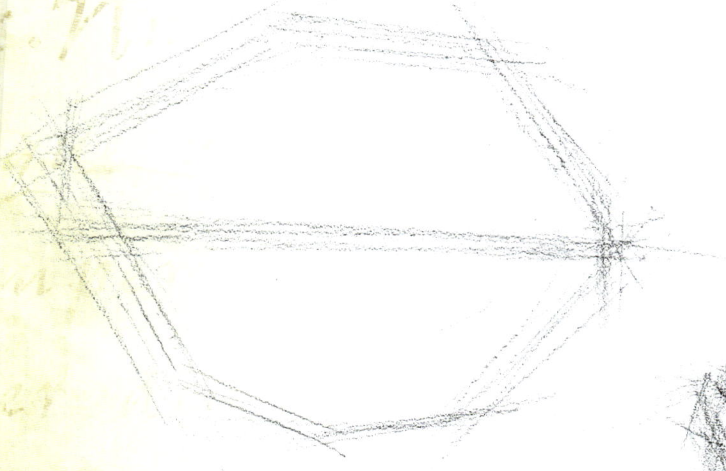

**1.** *Start with an accurate depiction of the eye socket. Build it with straight lines that stop when the shape changes direction. Use light line weight as you begin so there is no need to erase. With your divider, check the axis of the eye from corner to tear duct, and then draw.*

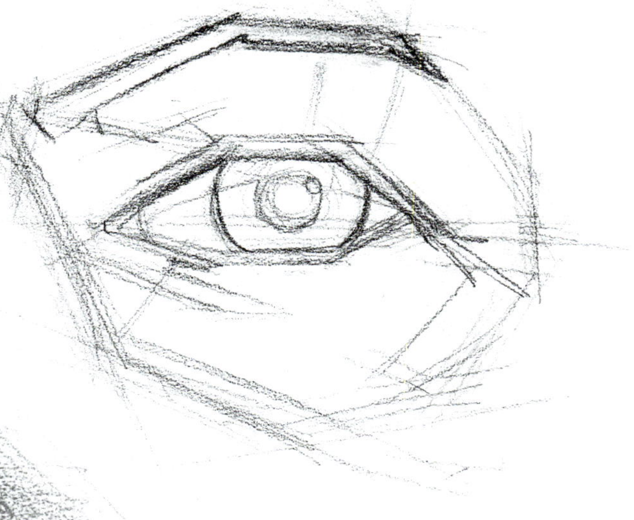

**2.** *Build your puzzle pieces around the eye first, closely analyzing their specific shapes. Start with the eyebrow and work your way to the pupil, shape by shape. As you establish the changes in value, you will reveal the shapes and planes. Notice the fold above the top eyelid. Make sure to place a lip on the bottom lid to show structure and form. Eclipse the iris by both the top and bottom lid.*

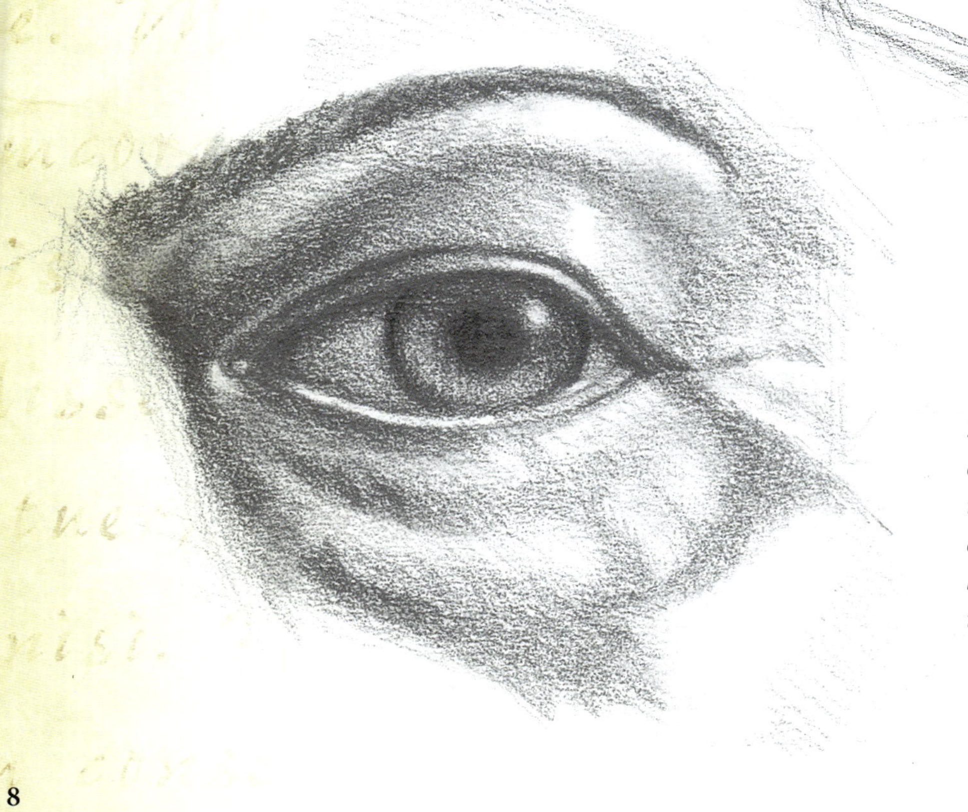

**3.** *When applying value, you are revealing the spherical form of the eyeball. Starting with your darks, gradually build the tone in accordance with your shapes. Look for soft and hard edges of each shadow. The reflection in the eye will be the lightest light. Be sure to apply enough even tone to reach all the values and create a sense of form.*

# NOSES

Noses must have proper structure and volume in order to "rise" from the face. Size and placement are crucial to a successful portrait. Just like people, noses come in many shapes and sizes. Many adjectives are used to describe noses, from "button" to "distinguished." Be true to your subject—see, observe, and draw.

**1.** *First block in the base of the nose; then map the angle of the nose and draw the bridge. Pay close attention to the angle and width of the bridge. Connect the top of the nose with the base, separating the side of the nose from the face. This creates a simplified shape of the nose.*

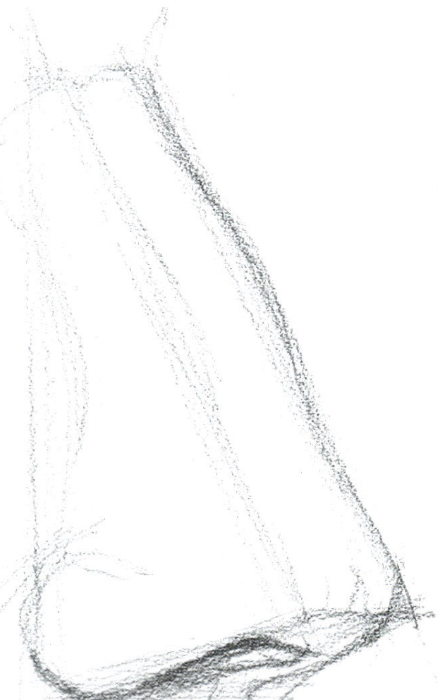

**2.** *Draw the nostril within the base of the nose. Make the transition from geometric to organic line to create a more complex shape. With variation in your line weight, suggest the concavities and convexities of the form.*

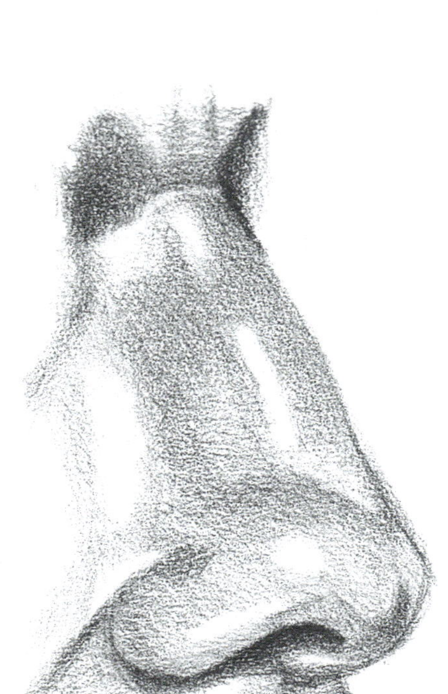

**3.** *Use even tone to separate the values of the nose. Your darkest darks will include the nostril and possibly parts of the eye socket. The lightest lights will be reflections only, so tone will cover everything else. Notice how the septum relates to the philtrum, the bridge to the forehead and eye sockets, and the side of the nose to the cheeks.*

## PRACTICING SELF-PORTRAITS

**One of the best ways to draw from life is to practice the art of the self-portrait. In figure courses, my students are instructed to draw themselves many times throughout the semester. Models aren't cheap, and friends won't always sit for you. Drawing from life is the most productive way to realize your portraiture skills. Photographs are easy to come by, but they're not nearly as beneficial. Mastery of a head's basic construction and measurements is most likely to occur when a three-dimensional form is right in front of you. Using mirrors and creativity, you can generate a variety of studio setups for your self-portraits. At the correct angle, a mirror at your side can reflect in a second mirror in front of you, allowing you to draw your profile. Rembrandt is revered for the many self-portraits he created. Draw yourself and practice the basic elements offered thus far.**

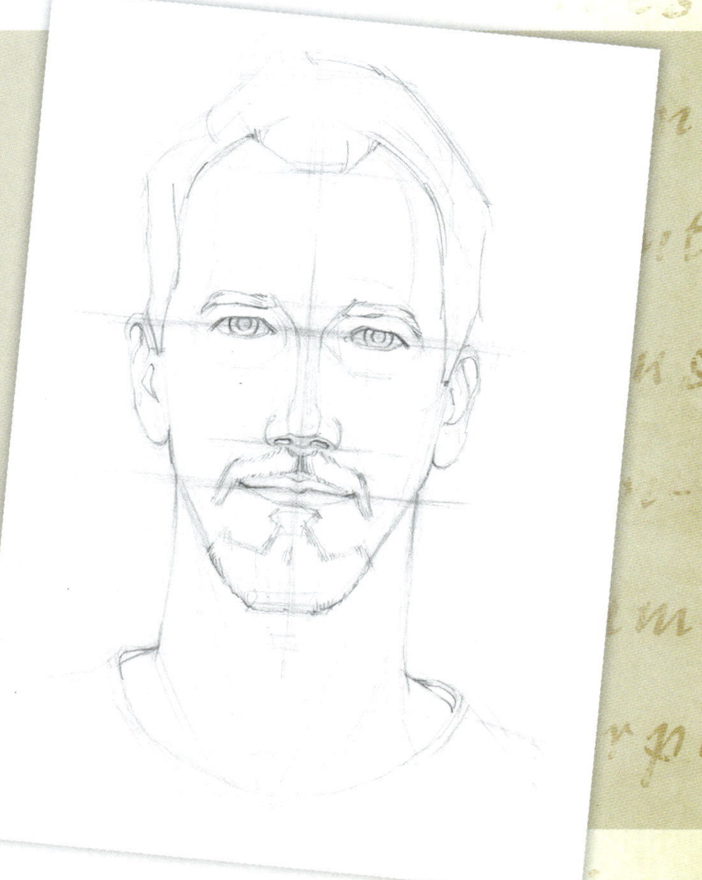

# Ears and Mouths

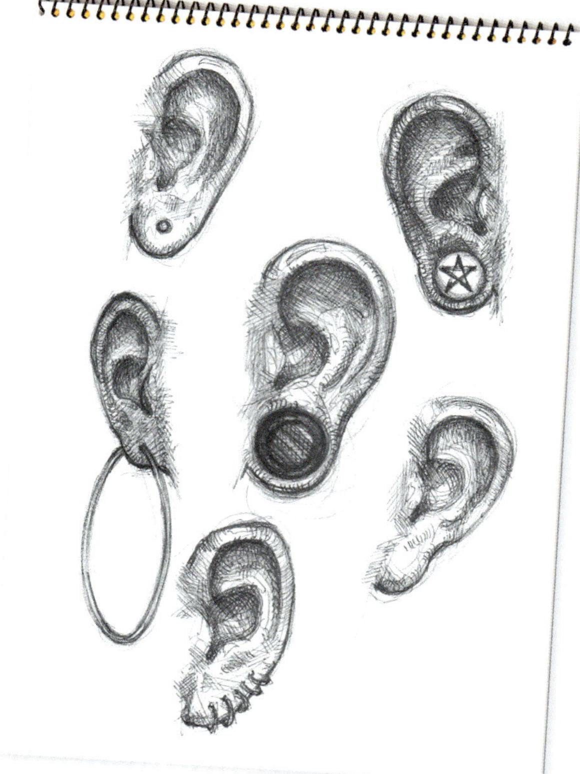

Ears and mouths are complex forms. Because they are rarely the focal point of a portrait, they are often simply suggested instead of truly rendered. However, you still need to draw them competently. A chain is only a strong as its weakest link. Good ears and mouths will leave no weak link in your drawings.

## Ears

Ears have many convexities and concavities. They can be obscured by hair or totally revealed. They can have accessories that are large and small, bright and dull. Some lobes are attached and others are not. Careful study of the particular ear or ears that you're drawing will help to reveal the unique qualities that are specific to the person you are drawing.

▶ **Ear Study** *Having a sketchbook and ballpoint pen on-the-go enabled me to complete these studies. Working as a VIP doorman at a club in Hollywood left me with plenty of time to draw while giving me access to a variety of subjects. On this particular night, ears and their many differences and accessories made for a worthwhile study.*

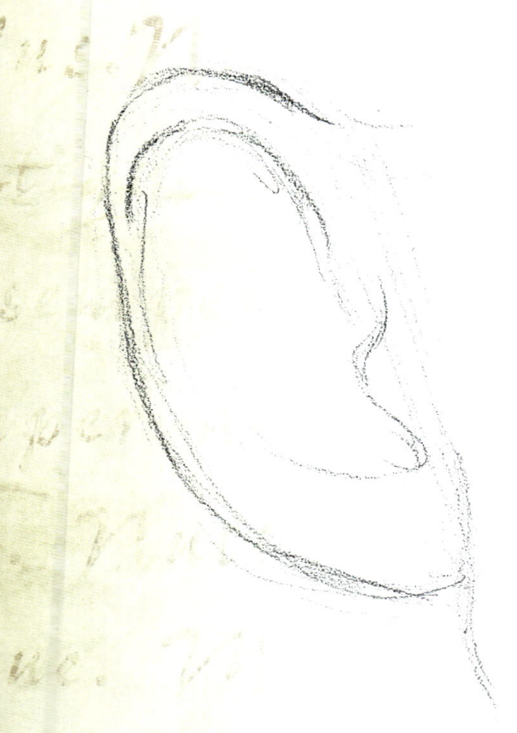

**1.** *Using light lines, draw the basic contour of the ear. Address the general interior shape that will contain the many variations of form.*

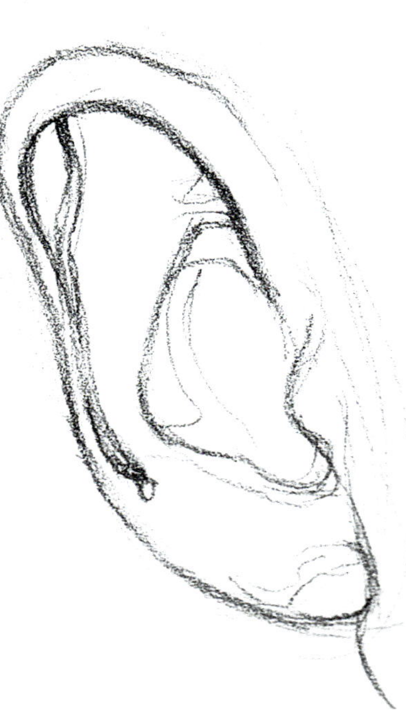

**2.** *Now move in with darker line weight and separate the shapes, following value patterns. Be sure to correspond your darker lines with your visual experience of value. The curve of your mark will show the concavity of center of the ear.*

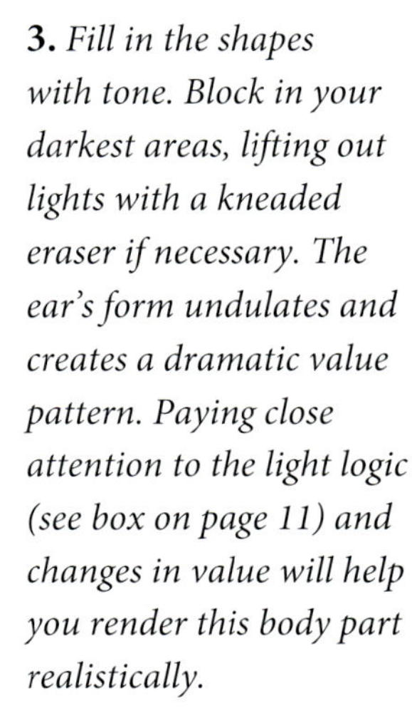

**3.** *Fill in the shapes with tone. Block in your darkest areas, lifting out lights with a kneaded eraser if necessary. The ear's form undulates and creates a dramatic value pattern. Paying close attention to the light logic (see box on page 11) and changes in value will help you render this body part realistically.*

# Mouth

When choosing a pose for a head drawing, the tradition is to have the mouth closed. Smiling lips and glaring teeth suggest a snapshot rather than a serious portrait. I've found that a pleasant look to the mouth is one with corners that are slightly turned up, communicating a timeless positivity. Smiles are also difficult for the sitter to hold. With this being said, there is no absolute and you should develop your own sensibilities as an artist.

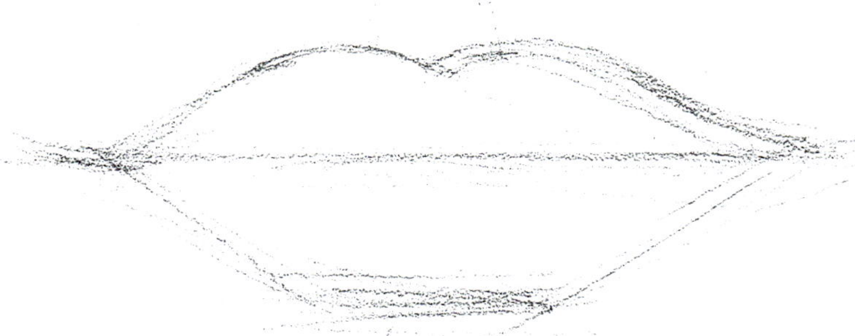

**1.** *First draw the shape of the upper lip. It receives less light, so it is darker and easier to translate. The bottom lip is then drawn in a simple shape using light, straight lines.*

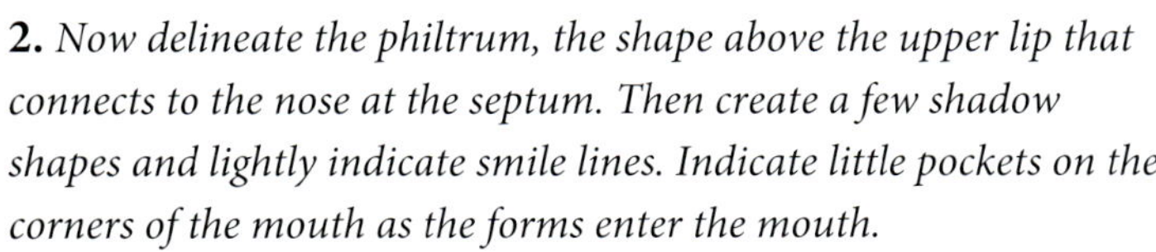

**2.** *Now delineate the philtrum, the shape above the upper lip that connects to the nose at the septum. Then create a few shadow shapes and lightly indicate smile lines. Indicate little pockets on the corners of the mouth as the forms enter the mouth.*

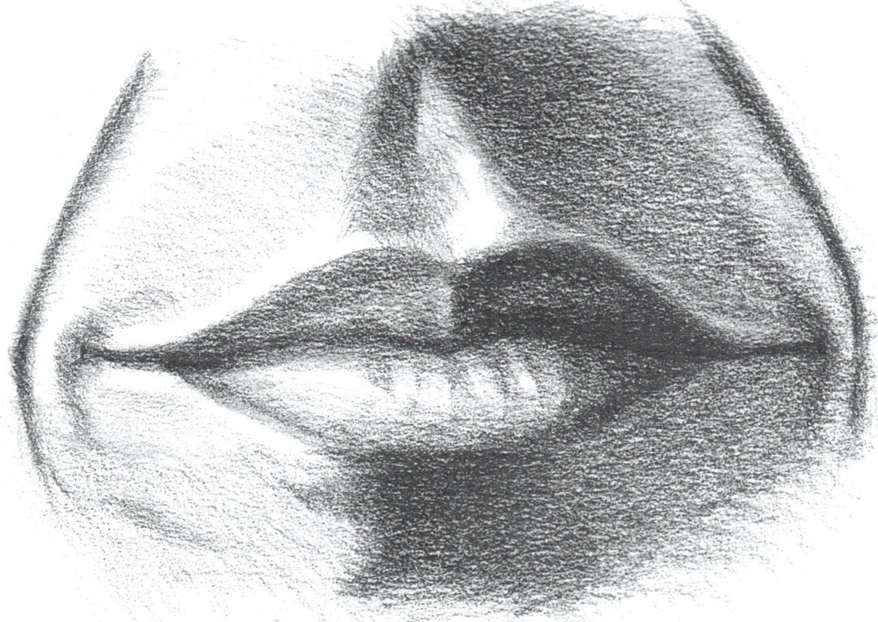

**3.** *Lips protrude from the face due to teeth beneath the surface. Because the philtrum is concave, roughly half is dark and half is light. The shadow shapes below the bottom lip, the right upper lip, and top right of the mouth are distinct and descriptive of the form of the mouth. Because of the way light falls from above, the upper lip is usually darker than the bottom lip. To finish, be sure to include the wrinkles and variations in the lip's surface.*

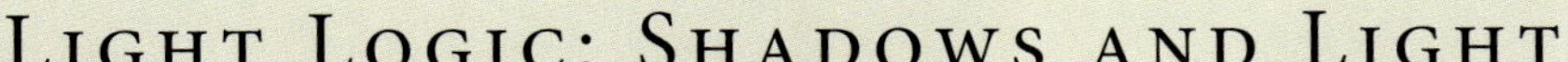

## Light Logic: Shadows and Light

***Light logic*** **refers to the way light logically falls onto objects. Representing light logic using tonal gradients will help you create the illusion of volume and form in a drawing. For example, a simple circle will become a sphere when you describe the light logic. Sometimes it's beneficial to push your values and increase contrast to intensify the illusion.**

**The anatomy of a sphere according to light logic includes the following elements: highlight, middle tone, shadow edge, core shadow, reflected light, contact shadow, and cast shadow. Accurately depicting these values creates the illusion of reality. Note: Keep the reflected light darker than the middle tones.**

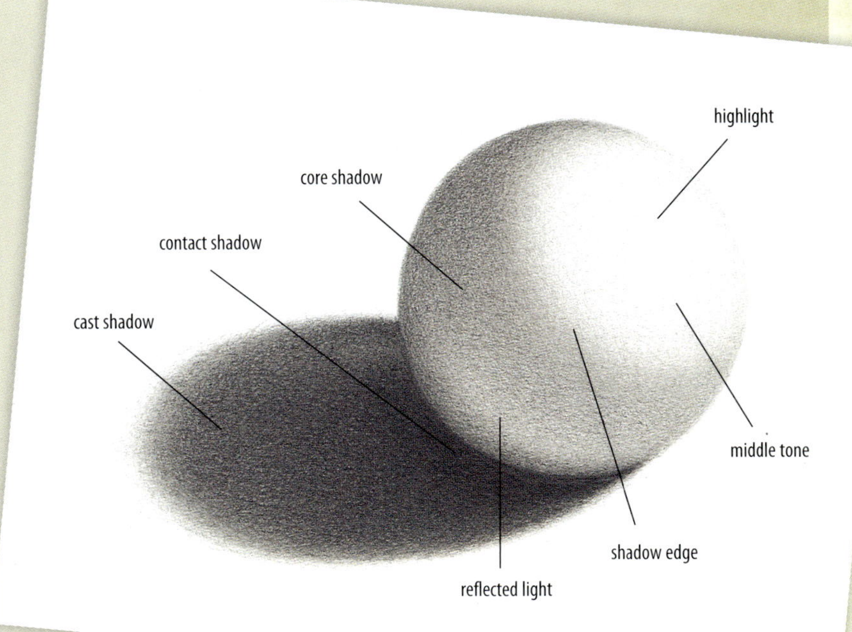

# Contour Drawing and Planar Analysis

**Contour drawing** and planar analysis are two exercises that will help improve your understanding of the head's form. Both are exercises in observation that are crucial parts of the drawing process as a whole. Each of these needs to be considered in the course of developing a drawing.

In a contour drawing, focus your line on the outside edges of forms and shapes. The line has character and its weight fluctuates in value. Spend most of your time looking at the model and not your paper. This will encourage you to record every nuance of each edge. Communicate value and texture with line only.

**1.** *Using a light line weight, sketch out a road map for drawing your subject. Place the eye line and mark the basic measurements. Develop the overall shape of the head and shoulders, and then focus your energy on the nuances of the edges.*

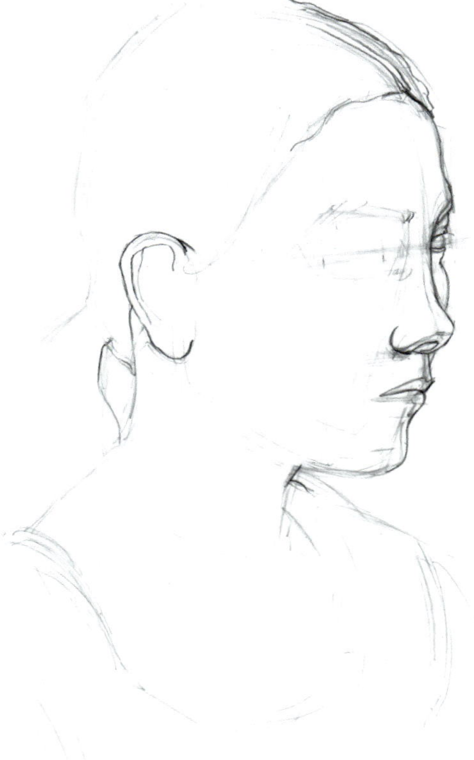

**2.** *Increase your observational skills and focus. Move in and out of the line weight; feel it and be it as you tap into emotion. Where forms overlap, use a darker line and push forms forward and backward. Overlap is crucial for developing a sense of space.*

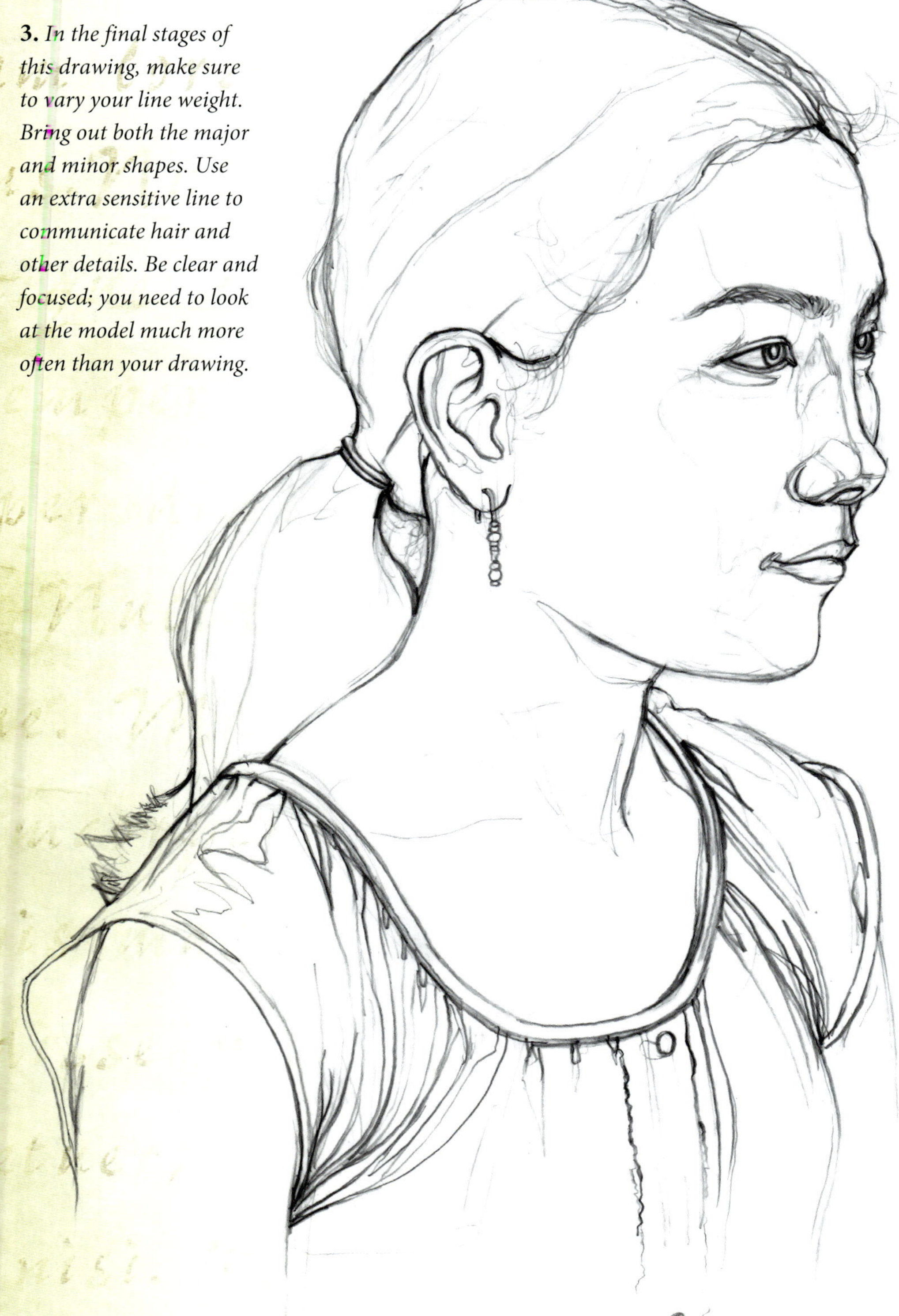

**3.** *In the final stages of this drawing, make sure to vary your line weight. Bring out both the major and minor shapes. Use an extra sensitive line to communicate hair and other details. Be clear and focused; you need to look at the model much more often than your drawing.*

Planar analysis is used to gain further understanding of the planes of the face. Treat your drawing as a sculpture. Think of this process as if you were carving the form from a block of stone, removing chunks with a chisel. The finished result will resemble a faceted diamond.

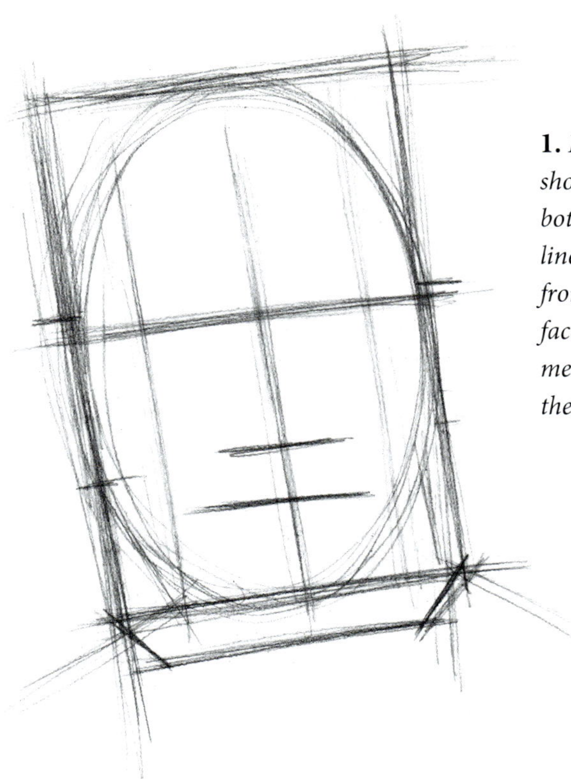

**1.** *Box in the head to show the front and bottom planes. Add lines to indicate the front and sides of the face. Then place basic measurement lines for the main features.*

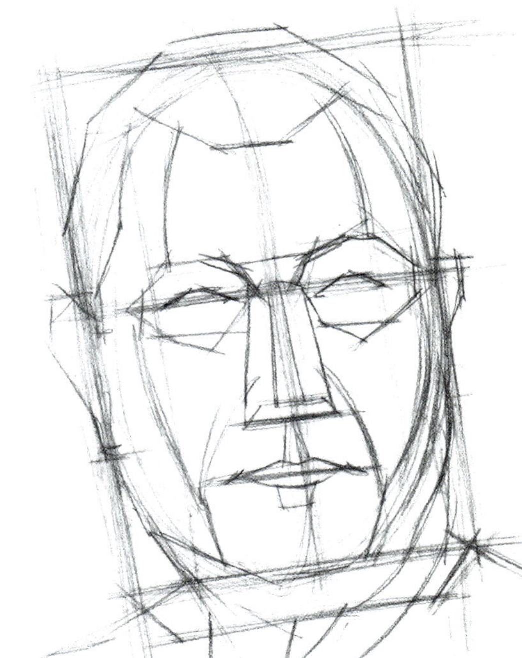

**2.** *Now chisel out the major planes of the face. Follow value patterns to help delineate the plane changes. Build the eye sockets, nose, and neck. Draw the hair shape, separating the face from the rest of the head.*

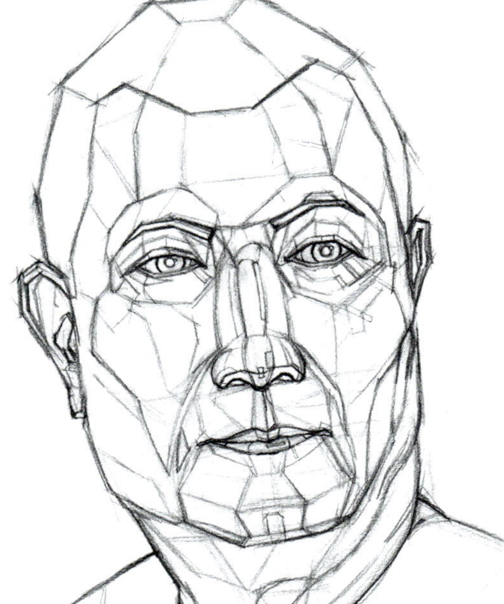

**3.** *Closely observe the variations in value. As a value on the face changes, so does the plane. Record the nuance of each individual plane and separate it from the major planes. Use your line weight to show the viewer what to look at first, second, and third. Note that minor planes should be lighter than major planes and masses.*

## Quick Sketches

**When you have a subject like my son, who was three months old at the time of this drawing, things become a little more difficult when drawing from life. Constantly on the move, an infant doesn't understand "hold still please." Focusing on the gesture helps. Make a gesture drawing by capturing the movement of the pose using many light lines and building from within. Then quickly attempt to establish the contour of the major shapes and solidify the sketch. This can be challenging but very rewarding.**

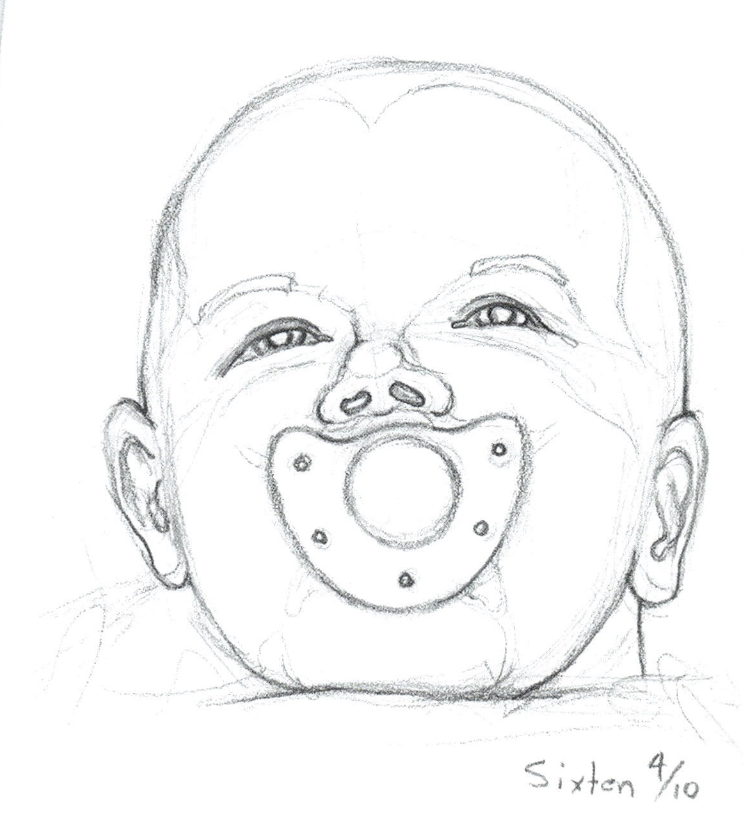

# Drawing Hair

**Drawing hair is easy and fun** if you use the right approach. Most people get caught up with the individual hairs and details without considering the simple shape first. If you treat all the hair as a whole, your effort will be painless. After indicating the simple shape of the hair, separate and block in the local values. Adding texture, detail, and character are the last steps in this process.

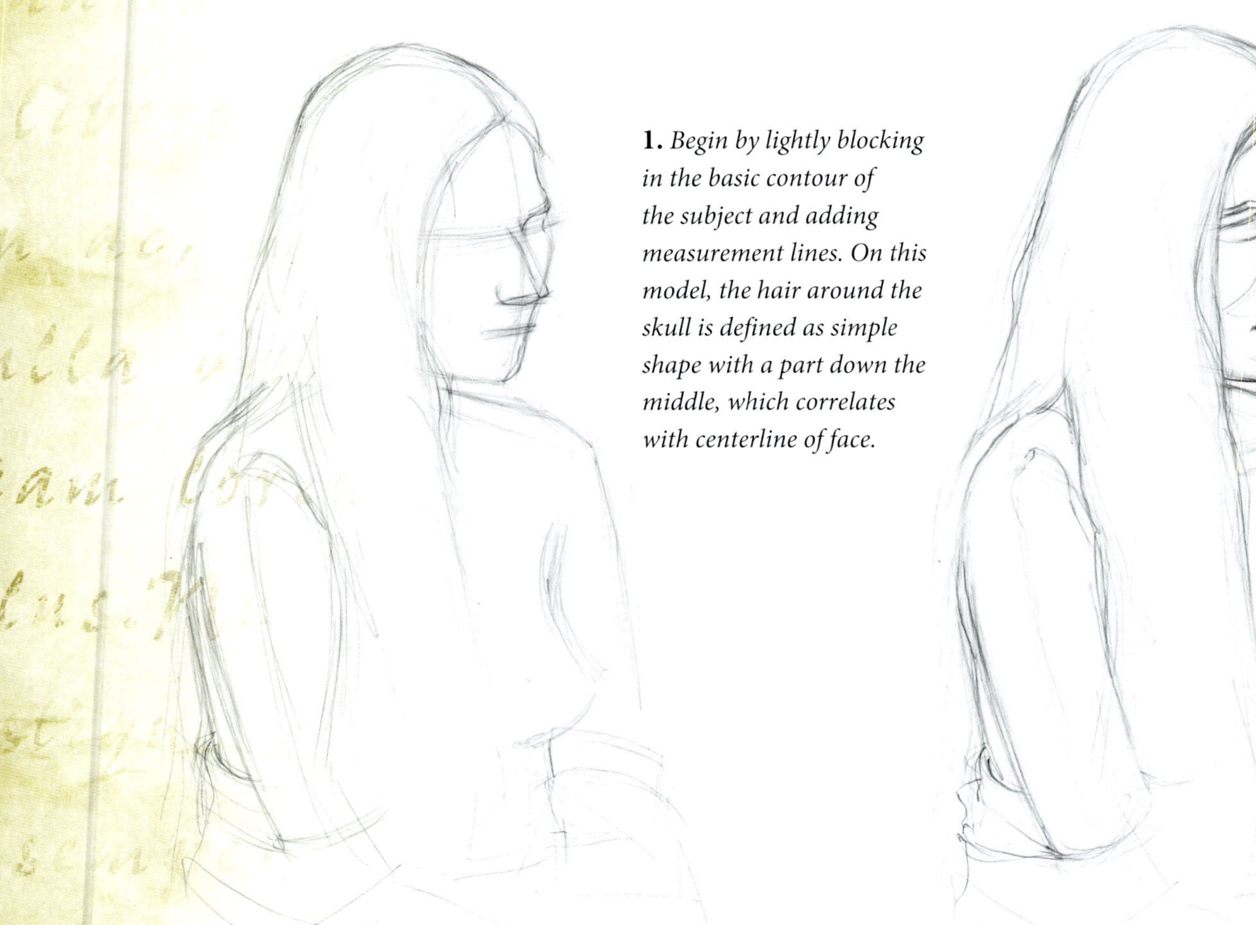

**1.** *Begin by lightly blocking in the basic contour of the subject and adding measurement lines. On this model, the hair around the skull is defined as simple shape with a part down the middle, which correlates with centerline of face.*

**2.** *Now increase your line weight and the value of the contour. Begin to draw shadow shapes and suggest value. Further define the hair shape and become slightly more specific and descriptive with your lines.*

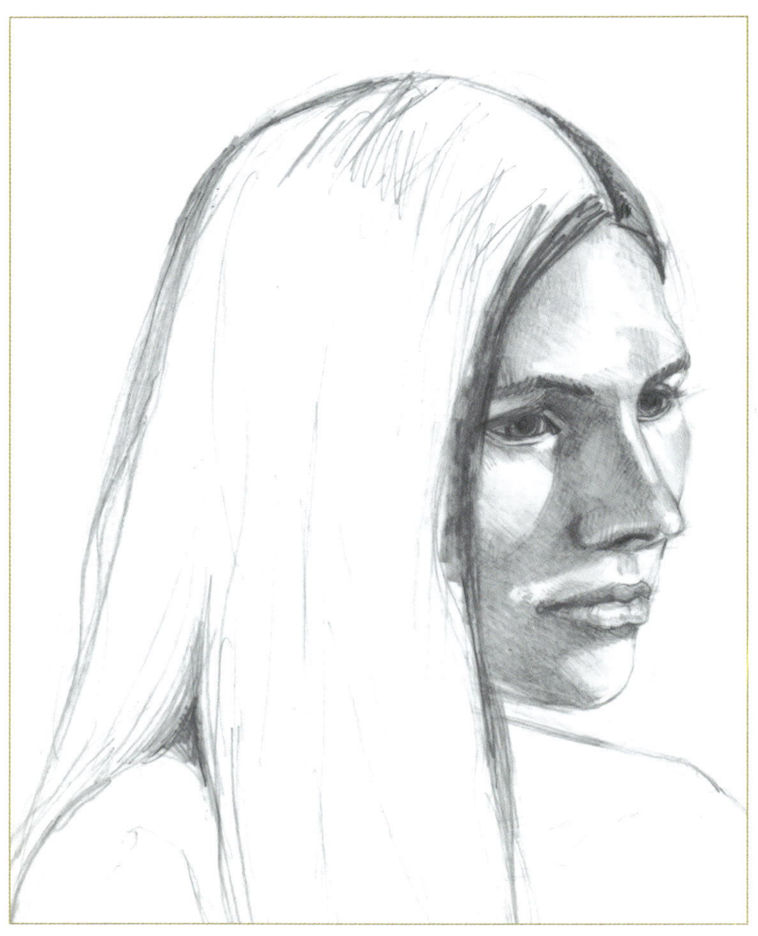

**3.** *Begin adding value to your shapes, starting with darks in the hair. The face is separated from the hair mass with tonal gradients. Use value to show where the hair parts and how it defines the face mask, separating it from the figure. Light lines within the hair help suggest direction and volume.*

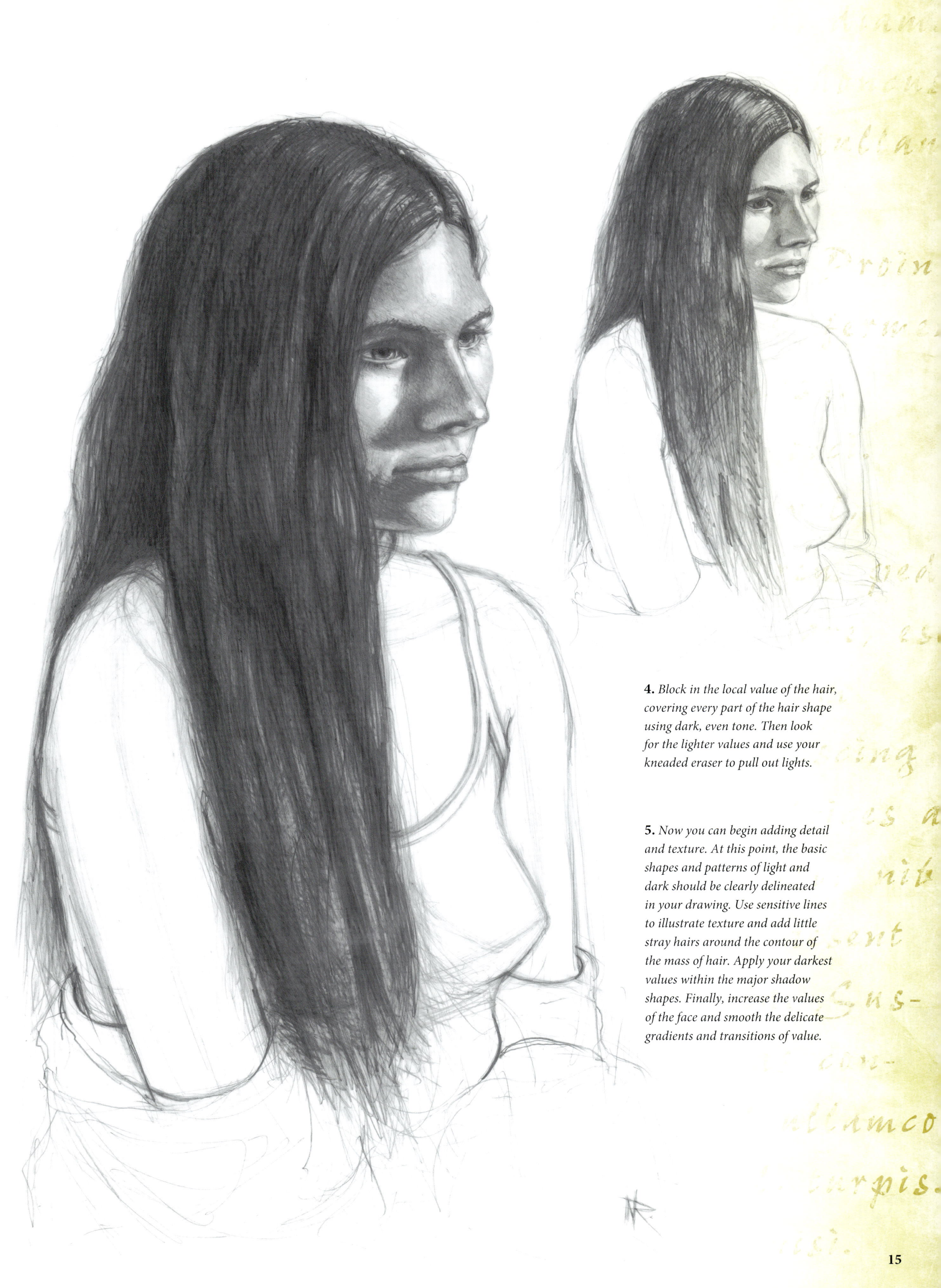

**4.** *Block in the local value of the hair, covering every part of the hair shape using dark, even tone. Then look for the lighter values and use your kneaded eraser to pull out lights.*

**5.** *Now you can begin adding detail and texture. At this point, the basic shapes and patterns of light and dark should be clearly delineated in your drawing. Use sensitive lines to illustrate texture and add little stray hairs around the contour of the mass of hair. Apply your darkest values within the major shadow shapes. Finally, increase the values of the face and smooth the delicate gradients and transitions of value.*

# Conveying Personality: Accessories

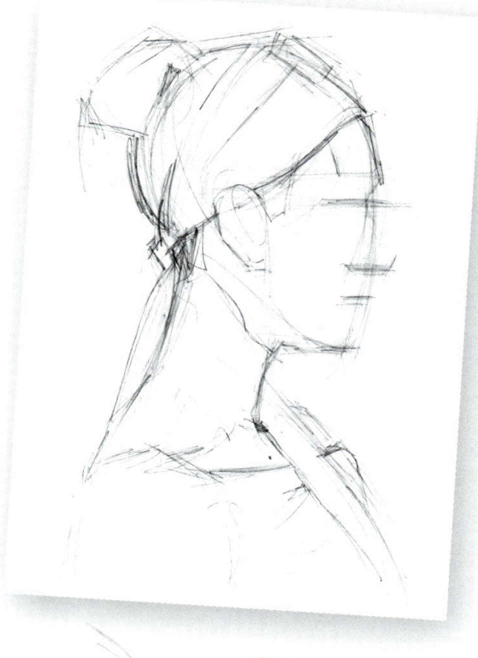

You might want to enhance your portrait drawings with accessories. Your job is not only to create a likeness, but also to suggest character and personality. With this profile in graphite, the head wrap accentuates the beauty and volumetric form of the cranial mass by containing the hair. The sunglasses and wrap set a casual mood for the drawing. They both communicate the sitter's personality and give a sense of time and place.

▶ **1.** *Begin the drawing with a general shape for the head. Mark the basic measurements for the eyes, nose, and mouth. Draw the planes of the base of the head under the mandible, from the chin to the ear. Lightly suggest the placement of the glasses and head wrap. The proper angle of the clavicle and shirt will suggest depth, so they must be calculated carefully for a profile view.*

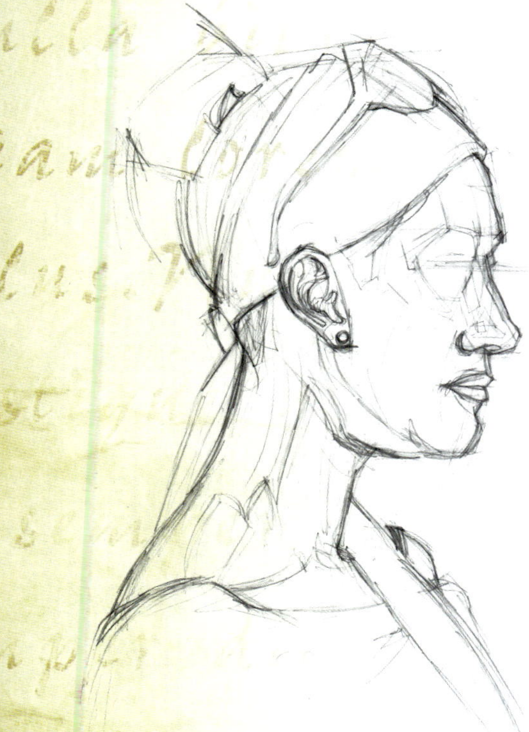

**2.** *When starting the eyes, build the eye socket first. Break down the ear into more complex and specific shapes. Map the angles of the lips, nose, and glasses, and begin separating shadow shapes and light shapes.*

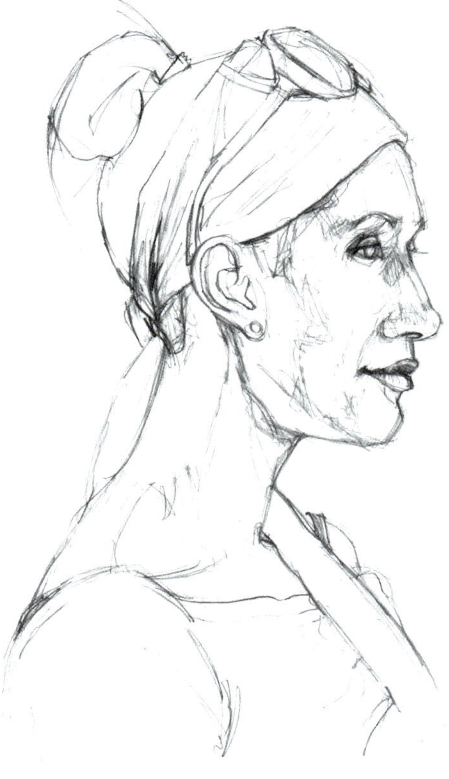

**3.** *Now focus on the quality of the contour marks and the variation of line weight throughout the drawing. Working in from the socket, develop the lids and eye. Then add the planes of the nose and shape of the nostril.*

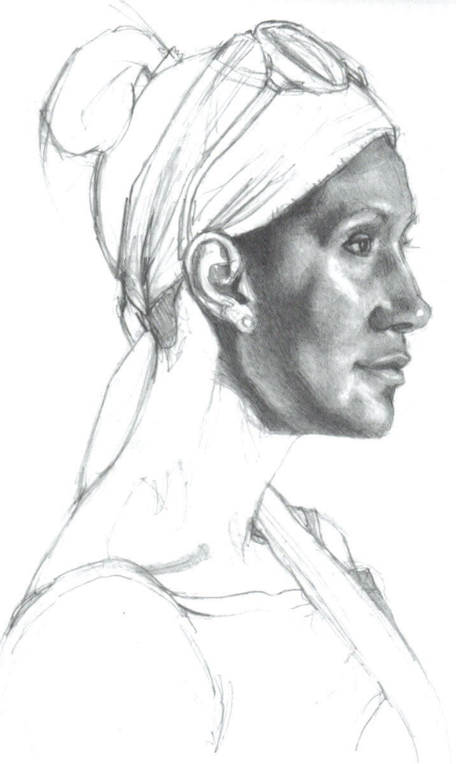

**4.** *Block in the local value for the flesh tone. For darker flesh tones, you might need several layers of graphite. Reflected light on the underside of the jaw must not be as light as the middle tones of the face. Reserve the darkest dark for the black hair.*

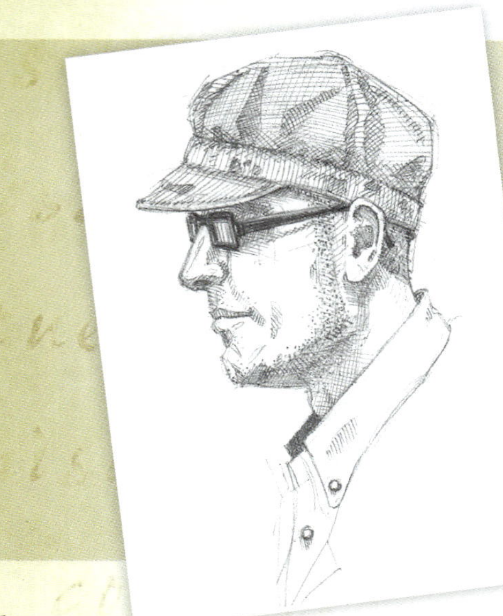

## Sketching a Likeness

**With my sketchbook and ballpoint pen, I have found that practicing on-the-go improves drawing skills, muscle memory, and actual memory. If people stand for you only for a few minutes (as in the case of this sketch), you can practice your memory of the subject when they walk away. And if they happen to come back for a moment, solidify and correct your drawing. With the accessories in this sketch, we don't even see the eyes of the subject, but one can still tell who the person is based on the head shape and personal wardrobe.**

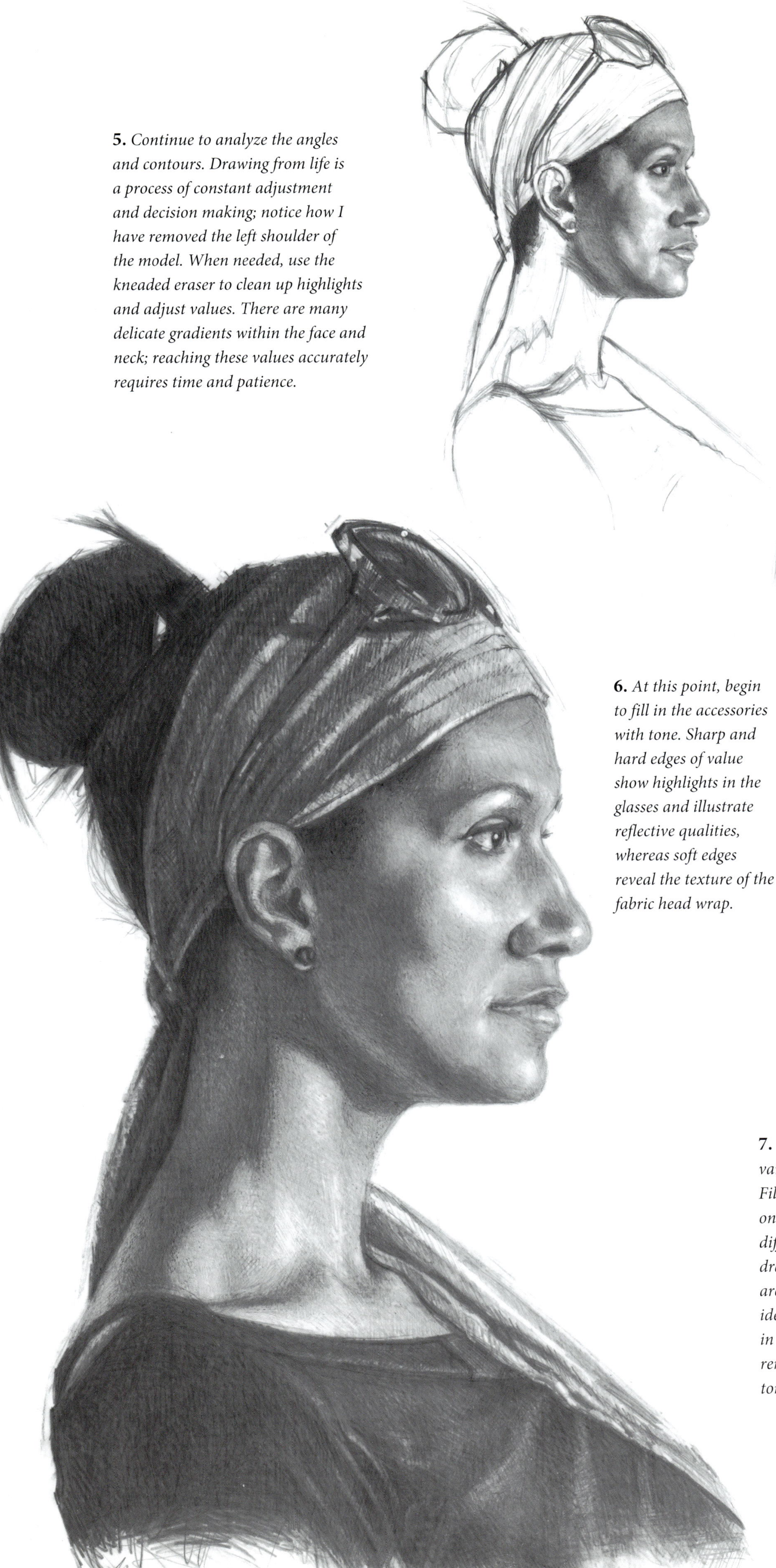

**5.** *Continue to analyze the angles and contours. Drawing from life is a process of constant adjustment and decision making; notice how I have removed the left shoulder of the model. When needed, use the kneaded eraser to clean up highlights and adjust values. There are many delicate gradients within the face and neck; reaching these values accurately requires time and patience.*

**6.** *At this point, begin to fill in the accessories with tone. Sharp and hard edges of value show highlights in the glasses and illustrate reflective qualities, whereas soft edges reveal the texture of the fabric head wrap.*

**7.** *Within the darkness of the hair, create slight variations to show the planes of the hair mass. Fill in the shirt with tone, catching the light on the folds of the shirt. Focus on showing the difference in the various textures within the drawing. Also, make sure the local value of each area is separate from the others and has its own identity. Careful attention to delicate gradients in the flesh tone will help you create a lifelike rendering. Make your final adjustments to the tones using a kneaded eraser.*

# Conveying Personality: Costume

**This frontal portrait** is character driven, so I choose to include the fishing hat, beard, and coat. Creating different personas for your models using costume elements can help keep things interesting. It's a good idea to spice up your portfolio with variety, showcasing your versatility with different body types, races, and characters.

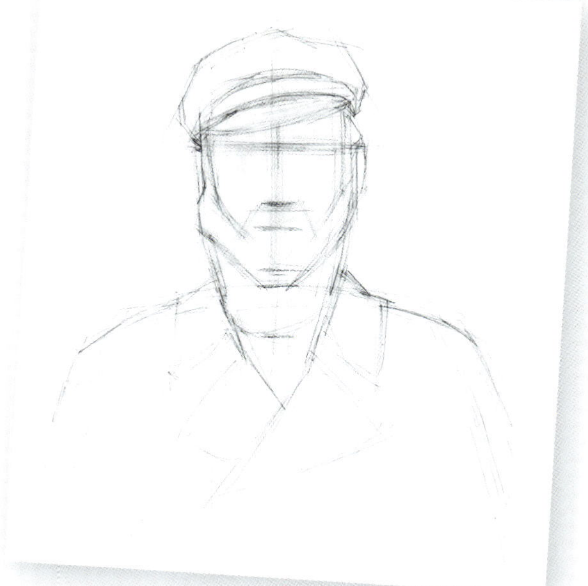

▶ **1.** *With a frontal portrait, notice the measurement cross in the center of the face. This cross combines the eye line and centerline. Because the model was standing and I was sitting during this portrait, the eye line is a little higher on the face than it would be from a straight-on view. With straight-line segments, use basic shapes to delineate the contour of the hat, face, beard, neck, and jacket.*

**2.** *Measure and check your angles early and continuously throughout the drawing process. The line in the beard on the chin designates a plane change from the front to bottom of the head. Chisel out the eye sockets and refine the contour and details, such as the buttons. Also, indicate a plane change at the base and bridge of the nose.*

**3.** *Separate shadows and variations in tone with light lines. Build the eyes using the shapes that surround them. At this point, begin to suggest value by the lightness or darkness of the contour lines.*

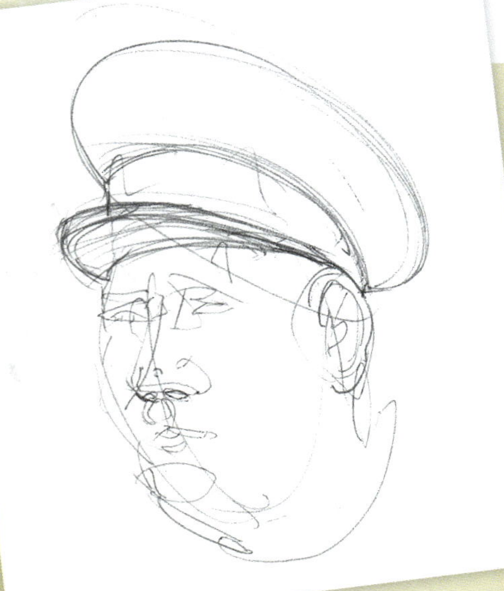

## Costume Elements

**In the sketch at left, the subject was walking by when his hat caught my eye—I just had to record it in my sketchbook. With this drawing, it was all about the ellipses and ovals. I quickly captured the centerline of the face and volume of the neck. The hat was such a treat to draw in conjunction with the rounded nature of his features. I had a minute or less to capture this gentleman, so in the true nature of the gesture, I never lifted my ballpoint pen off the page. I further developed the detail and structure of the hat after he had passed.**

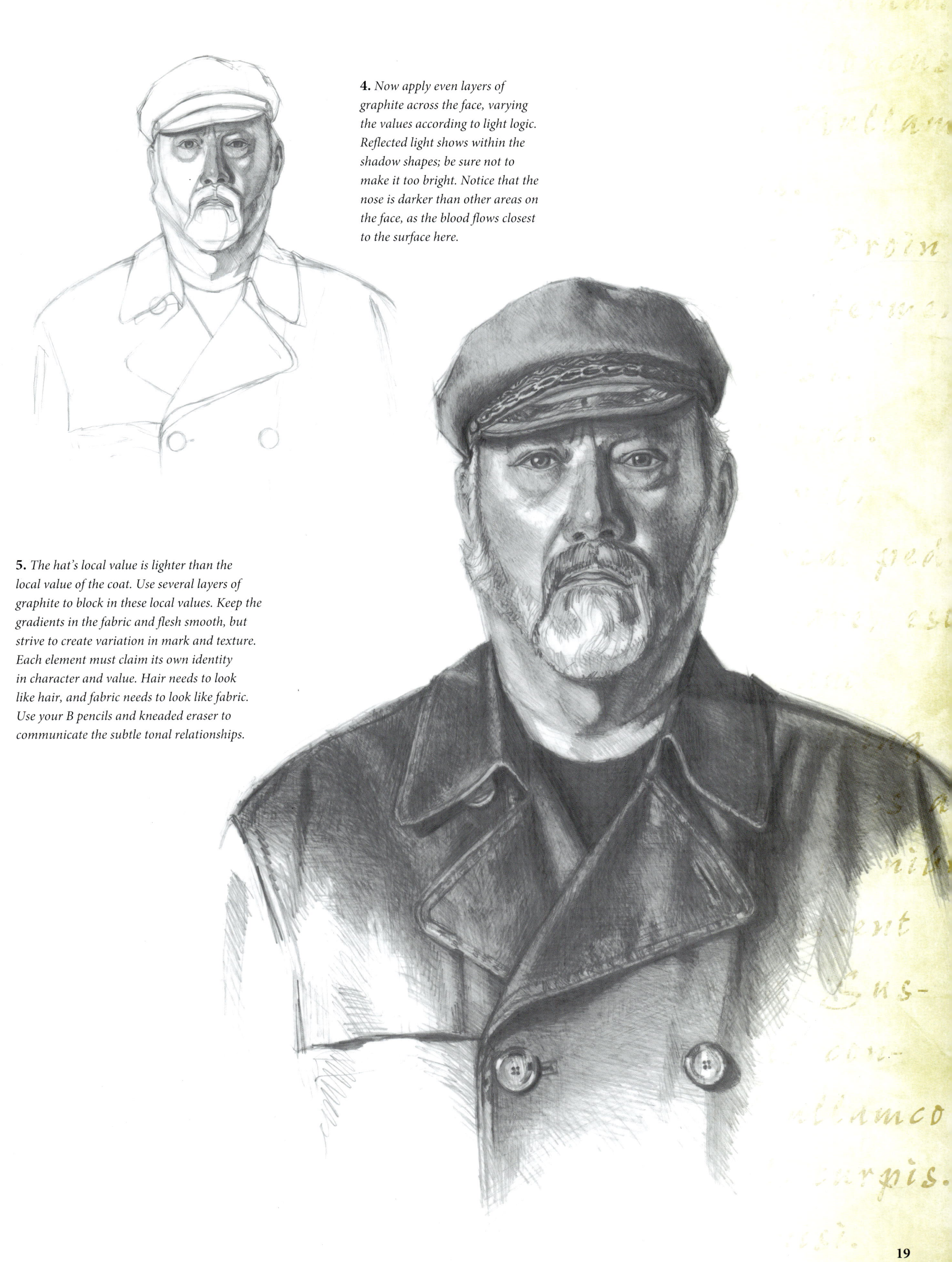

**4.** *Now apply even layers of graphite across the face, varying the values according to light logic. Reflected light shows within the shadow shapes; be sure not to make it too bright. Notice that the nose is darker than other areas on the face, as the blood flows closest to the surface here.*

**5.** *The hat's local value is lighter than the local value of the coat. Use several layers of graphite to block in these local values. Keep the gradients in the fabric and flesh smooth, but strive to create variation in mark and texture. Each element must claim its own identity in character and value. Hair needs to look like hair, and fabric needs to look like fabric. Use your B pencils and kneaded eraser to communicate the subtle tonal relationships.*

# Facial Expressions: 1

**Fear is an intense emotion** that causes a distinctive facial expression. The mouth is open and the eyes are transfixed. The forehead is scrunched, eyebrows are raised, and the shoulders are up. This is an emotion we can all relate to. When drawing this emotion, look at the basic facial measurements and how they change. With the jaw dropped, the mouth takes up a larger proportion of the face and changes shape; we can even see inside the mouth. The eyes open up and change shape as well. Good observational techniques will help you re-create this expression on paper.

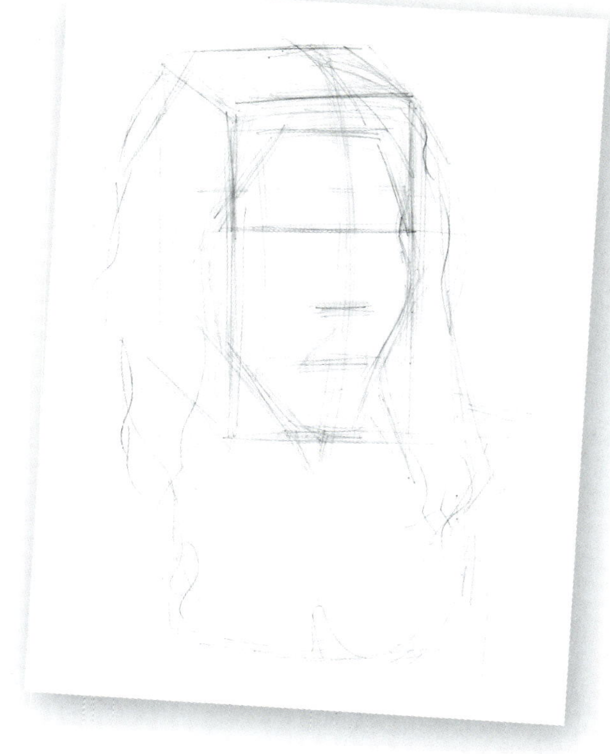

▶ **1.** *Start with a boxed head demonstrating its position. Draw a centerline through the face and cranial mass. Indicate the location of the eyes, nose, and mouth. Notice that the center of the mouth is lower than the general facial measurements.*

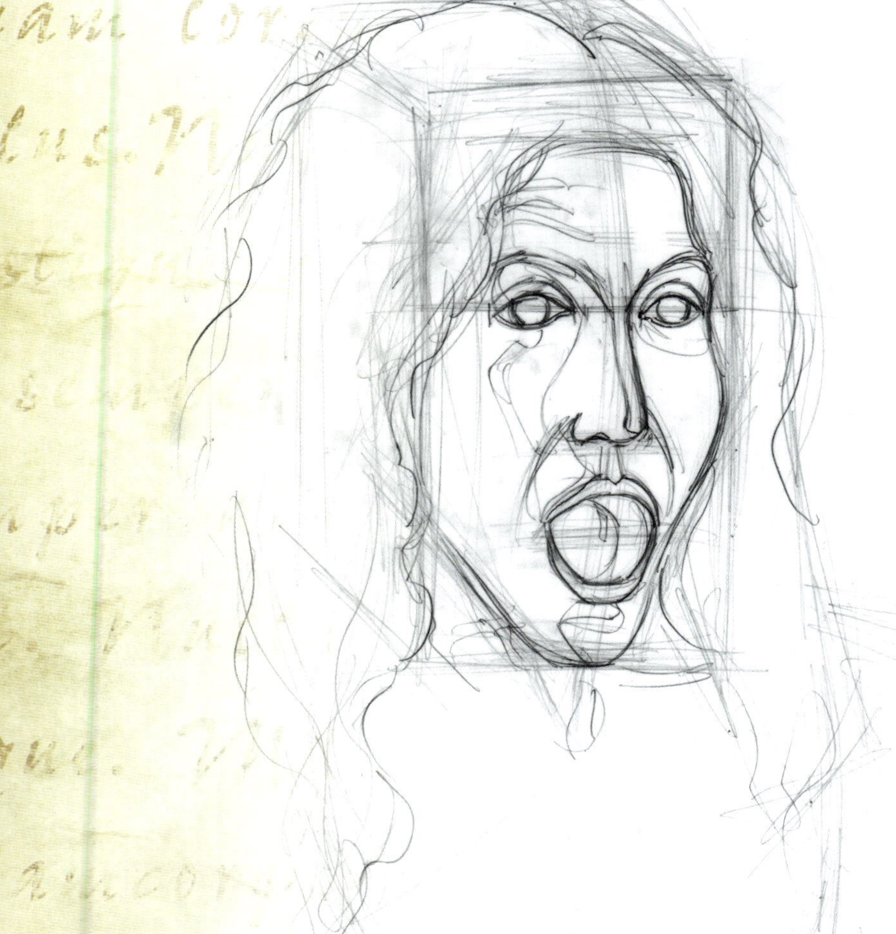

**2.** *Build the contours and solidify the basic shapes. Use a darker line weight for parts closer to you, and use a lighter line for parts farther away. Separate the shadow shapes and planes of the face with light lines.*

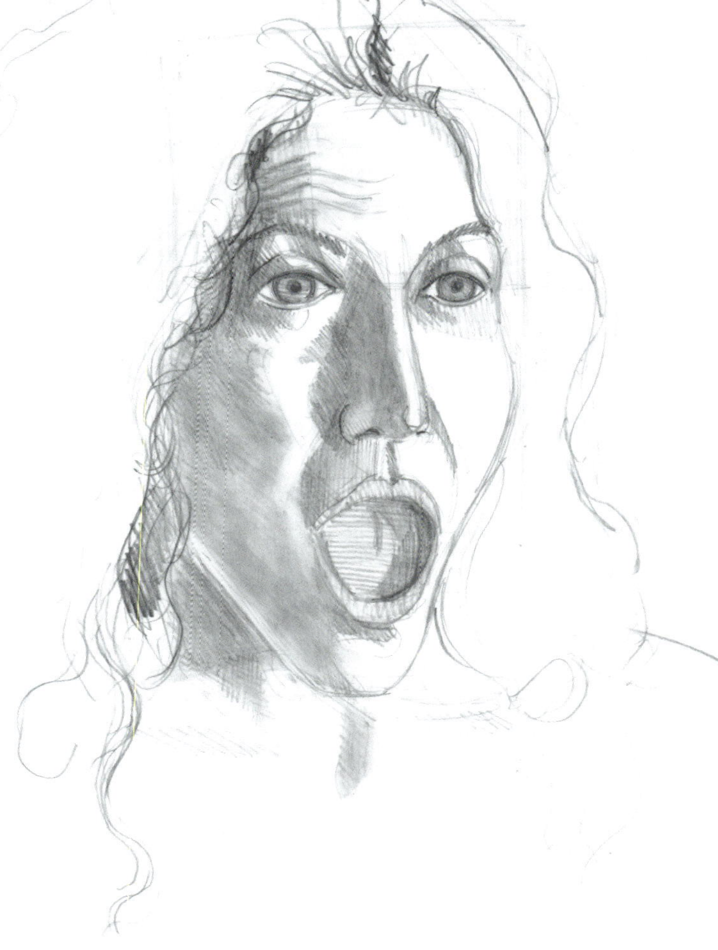

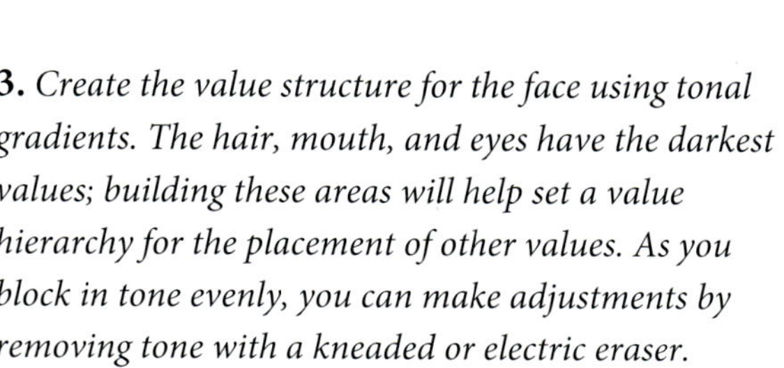

**3.** *Create the value structure for the face using tonal gradients. The hair, mouth, and eyes have the darkest values; building these areas will help set a value hierarchy for the placement of other values. As you block in tone evenly, you can make adjustments by removing tone with a kneaded or electric eraser.*

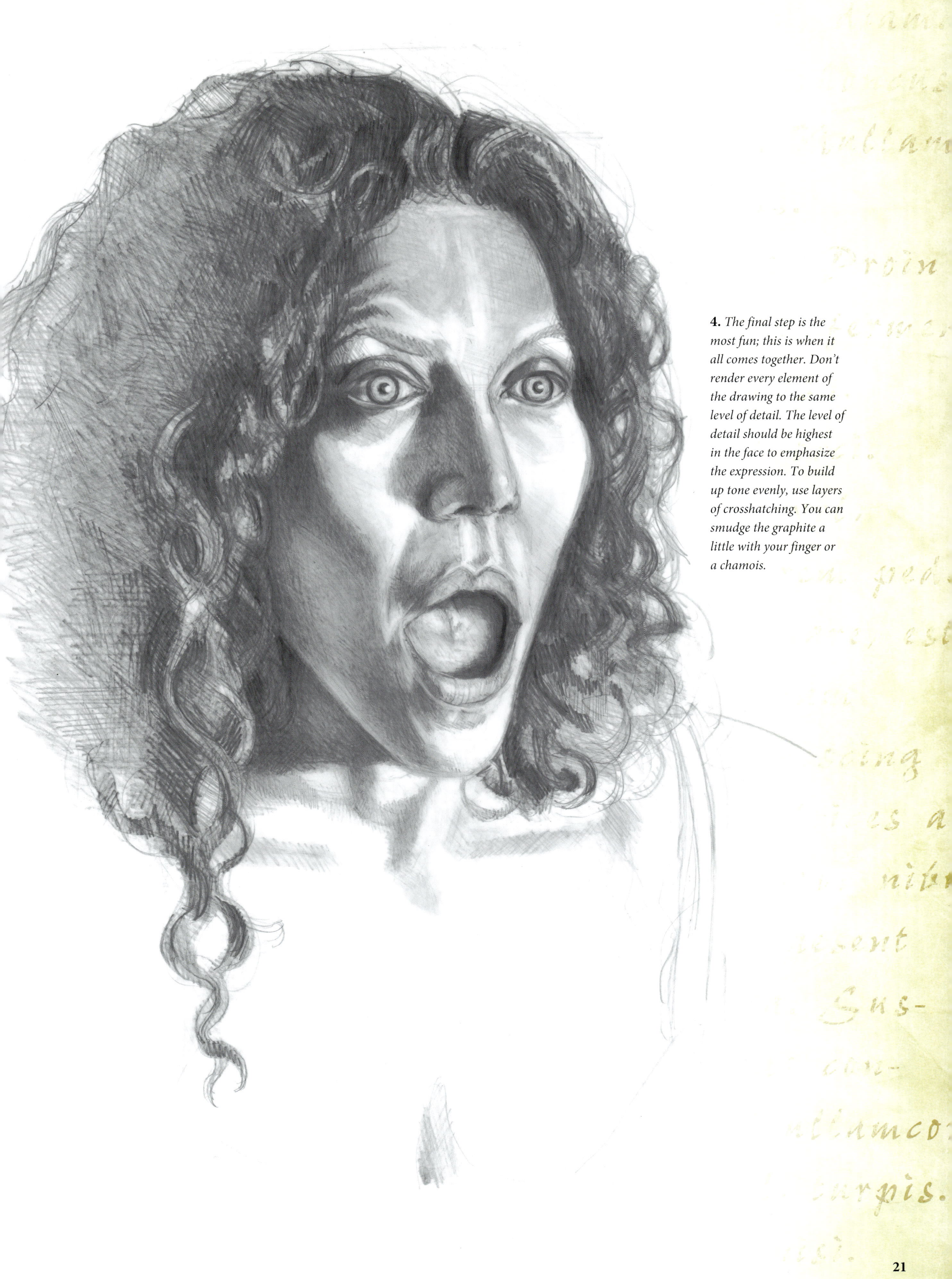

**4.** *The final step is the most fun; this is when it all comes together. Don't render every element of the drawing to the same level of detail. The level of detail should be highest in the face to emphasize the expression. To build up tone evenly, use layers of crosshatching. You can smudge the graphite a little with your finger or a chamois.*

# Facial Expressions: 2

**Communicating an emotion** in your head drawing doesn't always require an intense contortion of the face. With slight variations in your approach, you can change the viewer's perception of the subject. First consider your point of view and what it might say about the subject. Are we looking up at the sitter? This will exalt the subject and create a sense of reverence. Are we looking down at the sitter? This might suggest that the viewer is spying on the subject, getting a sneak peak. Even the slightest variation in point of view can change the way we look at a subject. The simple act of including a hand in your portrait will change its look and feel, as in Rodin's sculpture, *The Thinker.* Test out a number of poses and choose what is comfortable for you and your subject.

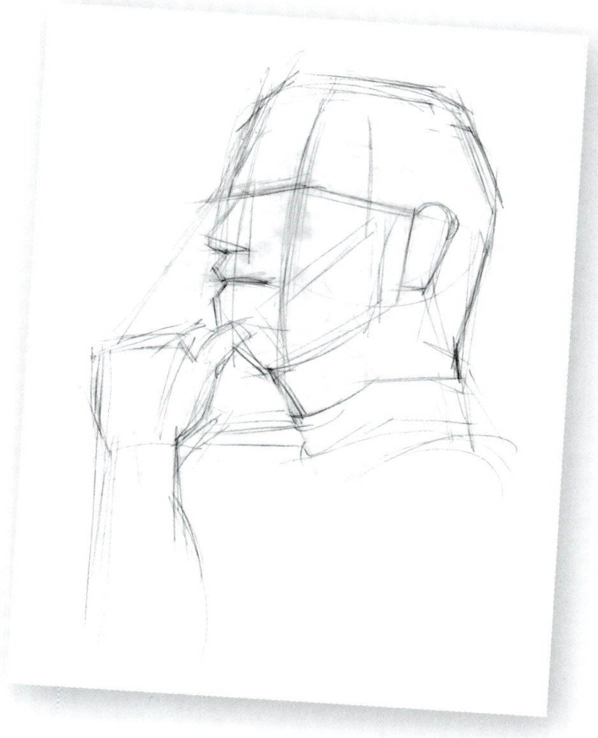

▶ **1.** *Begin with straight-line segments and carve out the major planes of the forms: the bottom, front, and side. Measure to analyze proportional changes when drawing from a new point of view. Use the angle check technique to help place and draw the hand.*

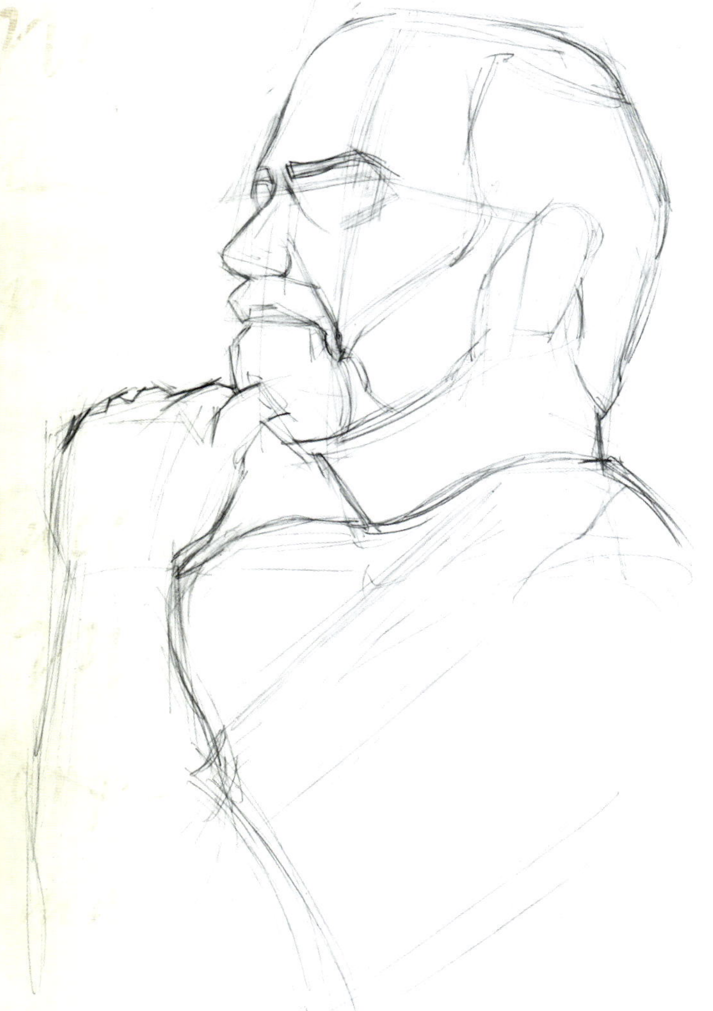

**2.** *Transition your lines from a geometric to an organic quality. Separate major forms with simple shapes, and contain areas within contours before jumping into detail. In a three-quarter view, remember that the far eye is hardly visible.*

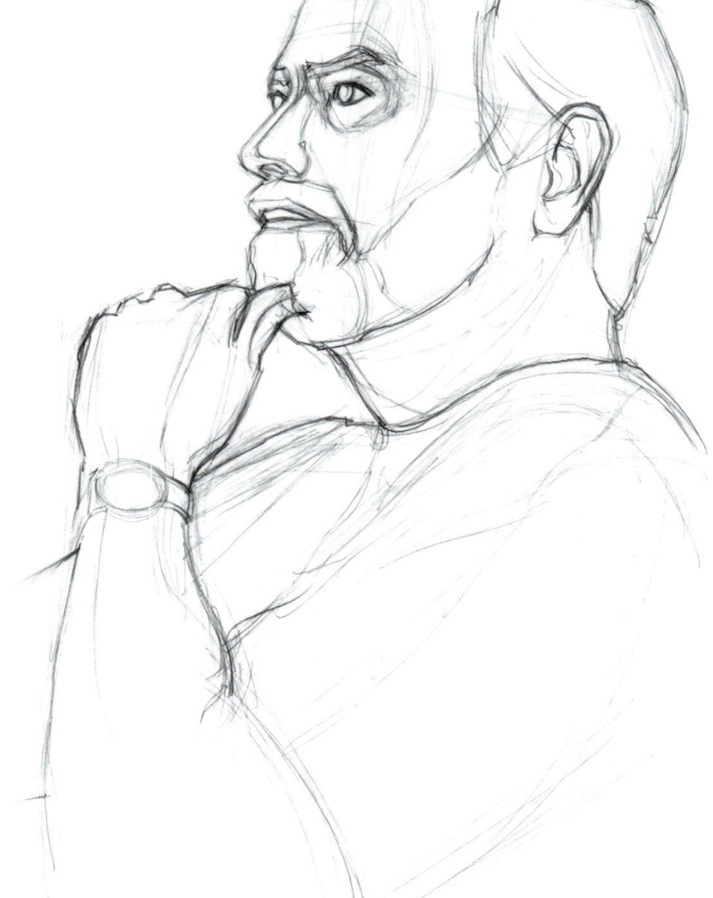

**3.** *Now that the major shapes of the head have been established, go into some detail. Break down the eye into the lids, iris, and tear duct. Separate the shadows from the light across the form, and then add accessories.*

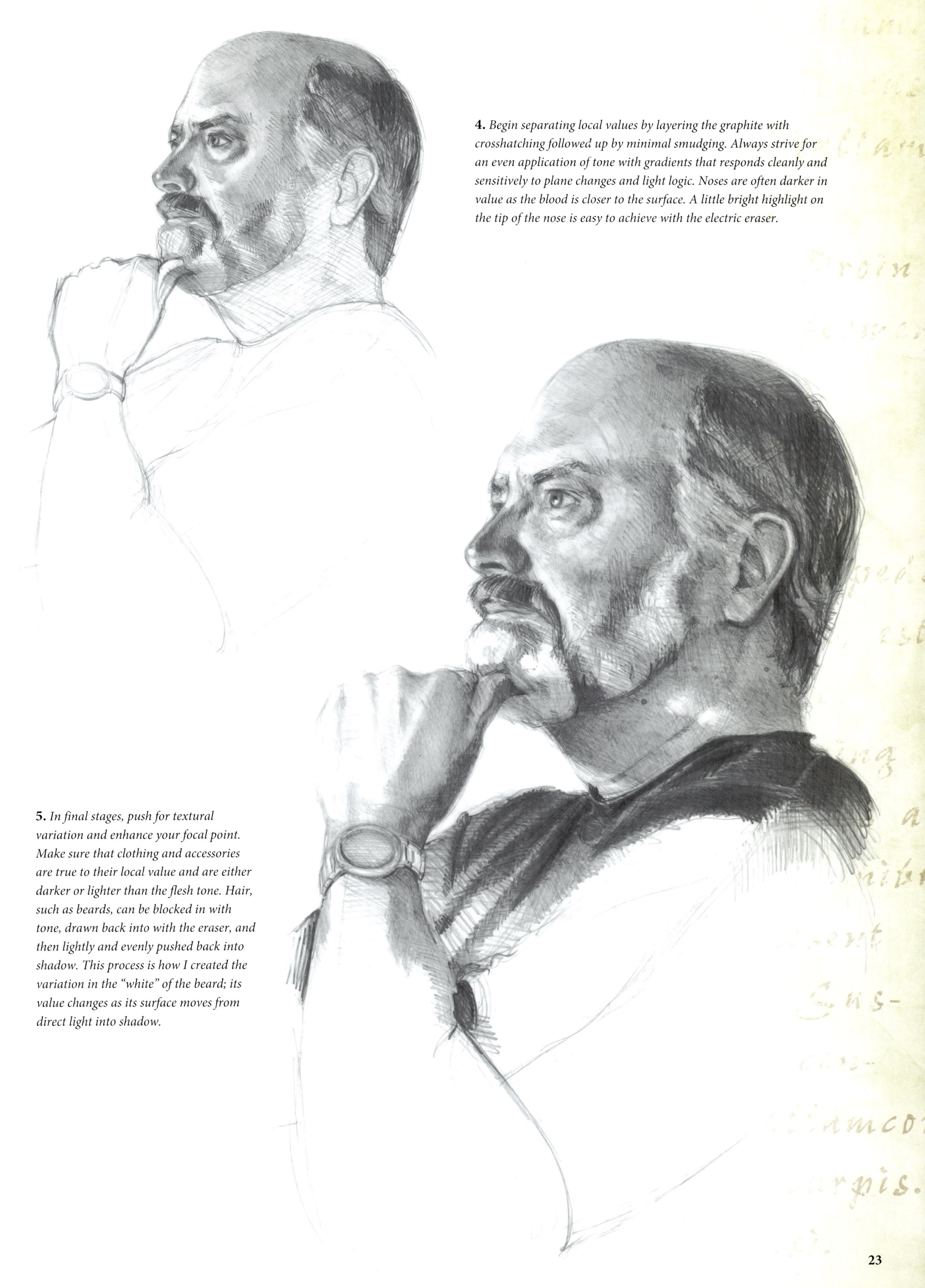

**4.** *Begin separating local values by layering the graphite with crosshatching followed up by minimal smudging. Always strive for an even application of tone with gradients that responds cleanly and sensitively to plane changes and light logic. Noses are often darker in value as the blood is closer to the surface. A little bright highlight on the tip of the nose is easy to achieve with the electric eraser.*

**5.** *In final stages, push for textural variation and enhance your focal point. Make sure that clothing and accessories are true to their local value and are either darker or lighter than the flesh tone. Hair, such as beards, can be blocked in with tone, drawn back into with the eraser, and then lightly and evenly pushed back into shadow. This process is how I created the variation in the "white" of the beard; its value changes as its surface moves from direct light into shadow.*

# Facial Expressions: 3

Drama is so fun to draw and can really give strength to a drawing. However, it is rare and difficult to find a model that can hold specific or contorted looks. The model I used for this portrait is an actress, performer, and figure model. When we started exploring the range of expressions she could create, I was impressed. Holding this look for hours under direct light is no easy task, and I am thankful to have had the opportunity to work with her. It's not about being comfortable—it's about creating a work of art. Working in your studio with a live model is a symbiotic relationship and a true joy.

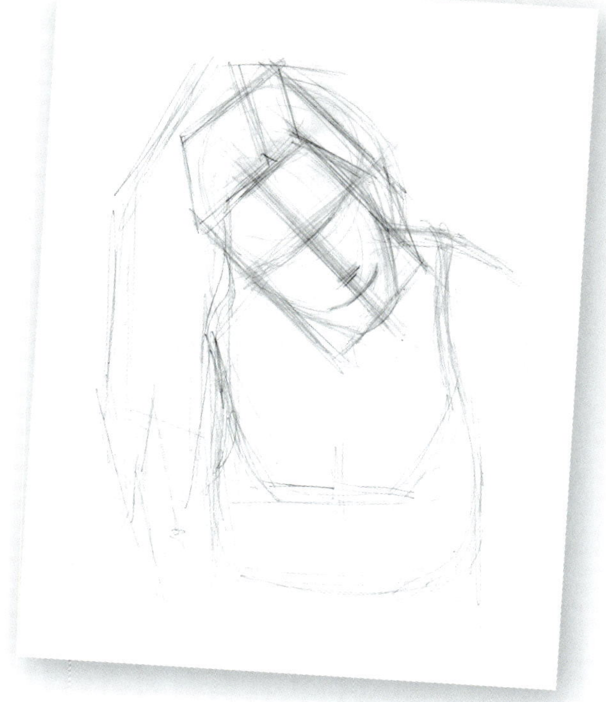

▶ **1.** *With a unique pose, it is vital to begin by drawing the "box" of the head in perspective. This will help you achieve volume and form while using an unfamiliar point of view. Check your angles, carefully ensuring that the viewer can truly understand the gesture of the head. Often beginners will fail to angle heads properly in this position. Use light construction lines to define other masses around the head. Then place measurements for the eyes, nose, and mouth.*

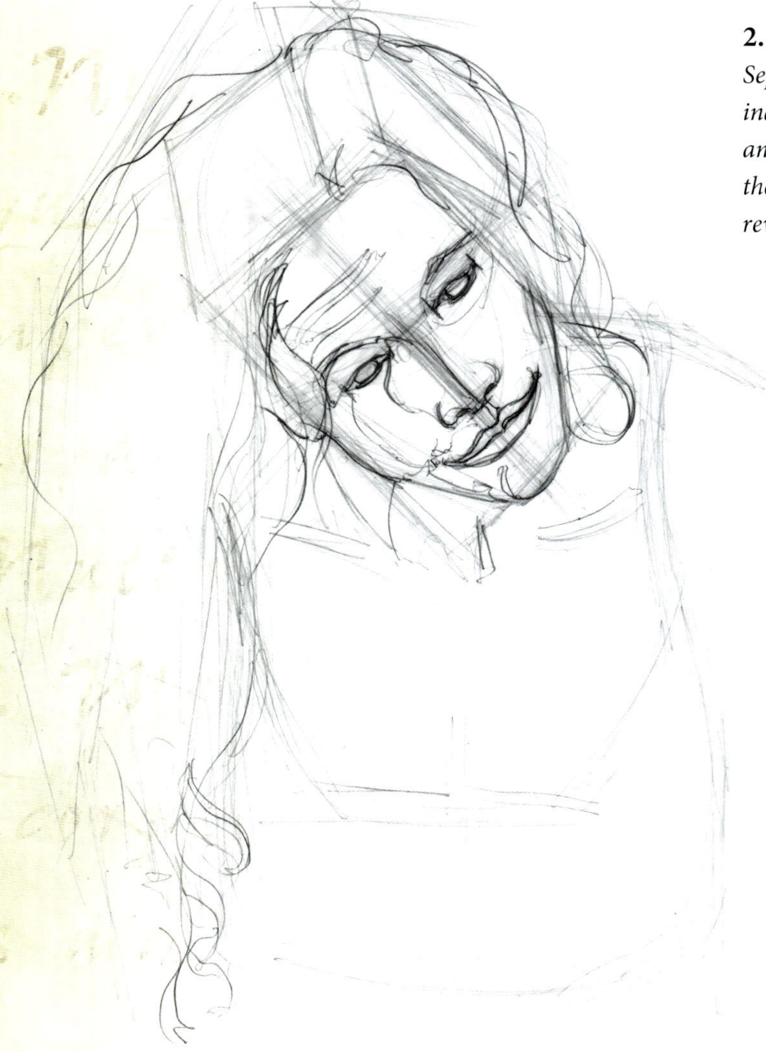

**2.** *Next, break down and establish the facial features. Separate light and shadow patterns with line. Then indicate the location and direction of the clavicles, and construct the pit of the neck and shoulders. Notice the curve of the strap and how its cross-contour mark reveals form.*

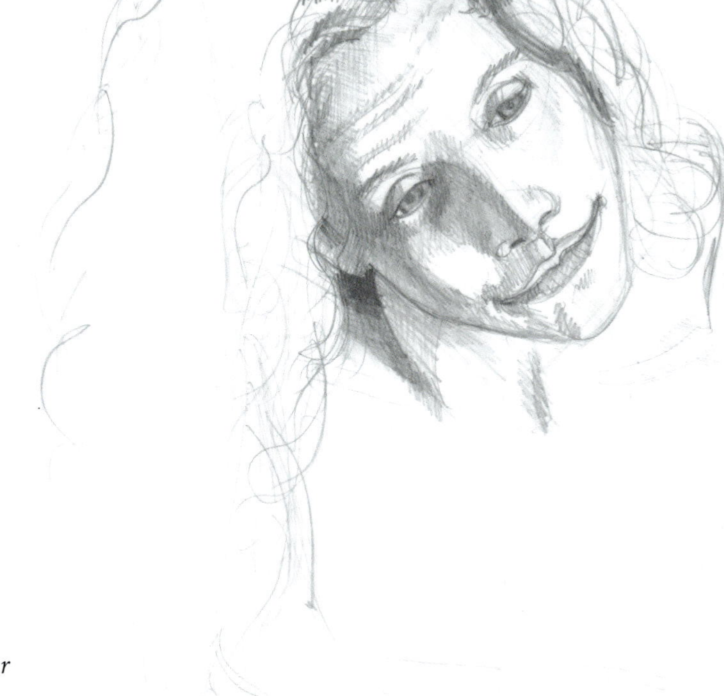

**3.** *Starting with the darkest dark will help set the stage for the other values. In this drawing, the darkest dark is under the ear. Once you apply this, separate the darker side of the face from the lighter side using light tone. Proper tones illustrate the connection of the head to the neck, as well as the neck to the shoulders.*

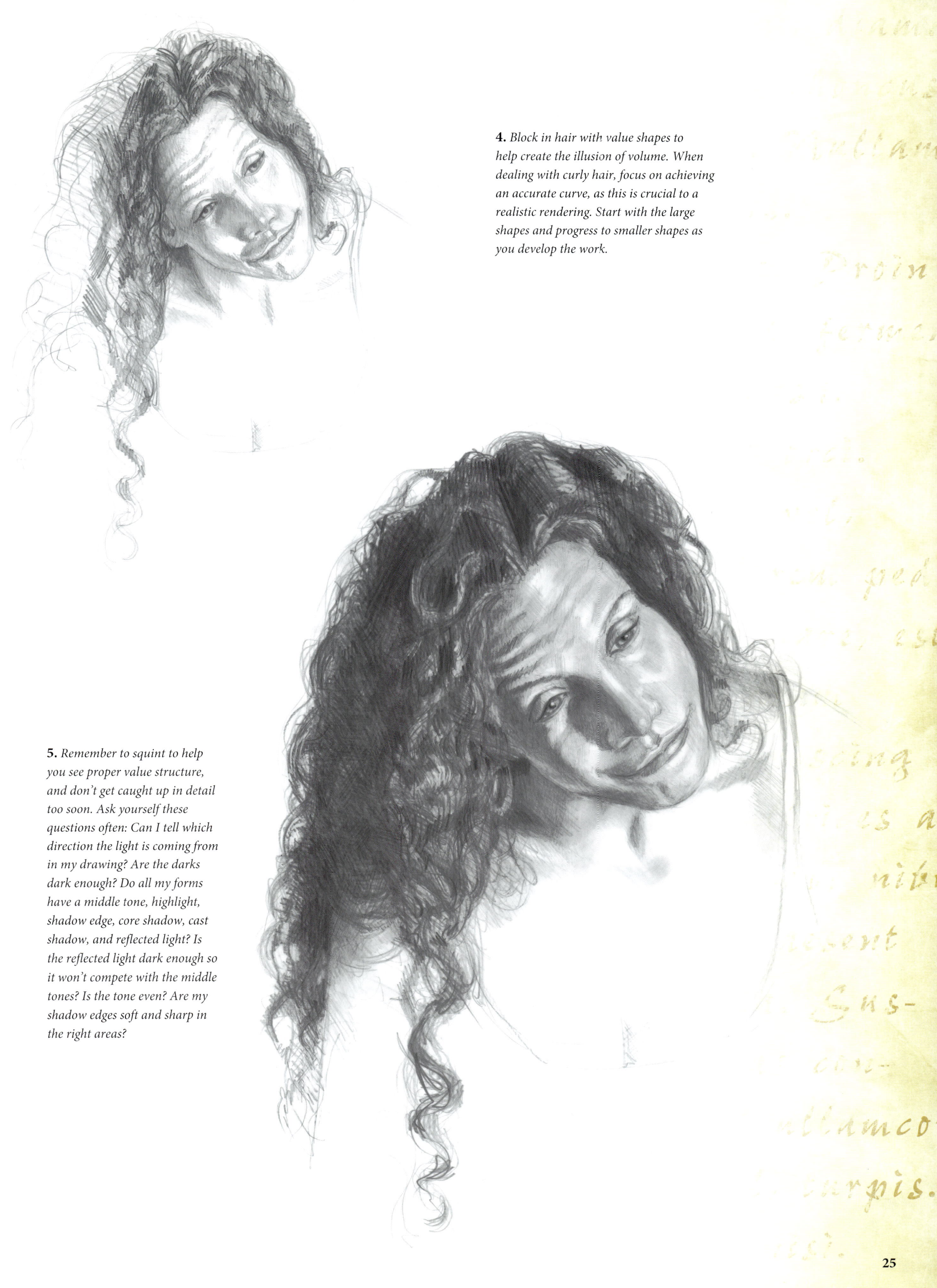

**4.** *Block in hair with value shapes to help create the illusion of volume. When dealing with curly hair, focus on achieving an accurate curve, as this is crucial to a realistic rendering. Start with the large shapes and progress to smaller shapes as you develop the work.*

**5.** *Remember to squint to help you see proper value structure, and don't get caught up in detail too soon. Ask yourself these questions often: Can I tell which direction the light is coming from in my drawing? Are the darks dark enough? Do all my forms have a middle tone, highlight, shadow edge, core shadow, cast shadow, and reflected light? Is the reflected light dark enough so it won't compete with the middle tones? Is the tone even? Are my shadow edges soft and sharp in the right areas?*

# Additive and Subtractive Charcoal

**Using an additive and subtractive** charcoal technique is quicker than rendering with graphite, and it can help you better understand value. Charcoal creates a dramatic and expressive result and can produce a dark black tone, which gives a finished piece plenty of punch. It also can be very smooth when smeared, producing subtle tonal gradients. And charcoal can also be layered and hatched for a more textured look. In this particular approach, apply charcoal to the paper and remove it with an eraser to refine your shapes and create form. Switch back and forth between charcoal and the eraser until you achieve your desired result.

▶ **1.** *First, tone the white drawing paper by rubbing over the surface with a stick of charcoal and smearing it with a chamois. I toned this paper with compressed charcoal, which produces a broad and slightly uneven tone. If you tone the paper with vine charcoal, you can begin your drawing with a more even tone. You can also choose to either tape the edges of your picture plane or leave them untaped for a more organic edge, as in this drawing.*

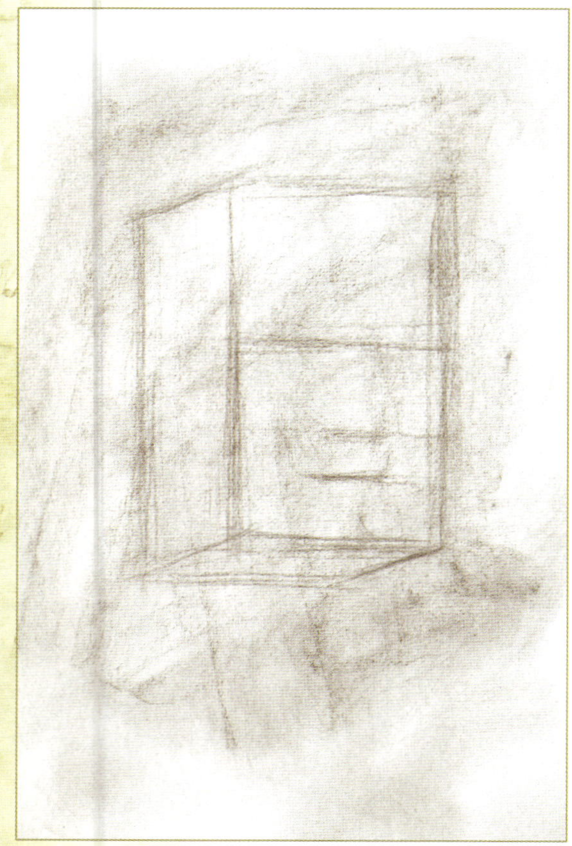

**2.** *With a stick of vine charcoal, box in the head to show the major planes and orient its place in space. Measure and mark the location of the eyes, nose, and mouth. We begin with vine charcoal because it is temporal and mistakes can be wiped away with the touch of a finger.*

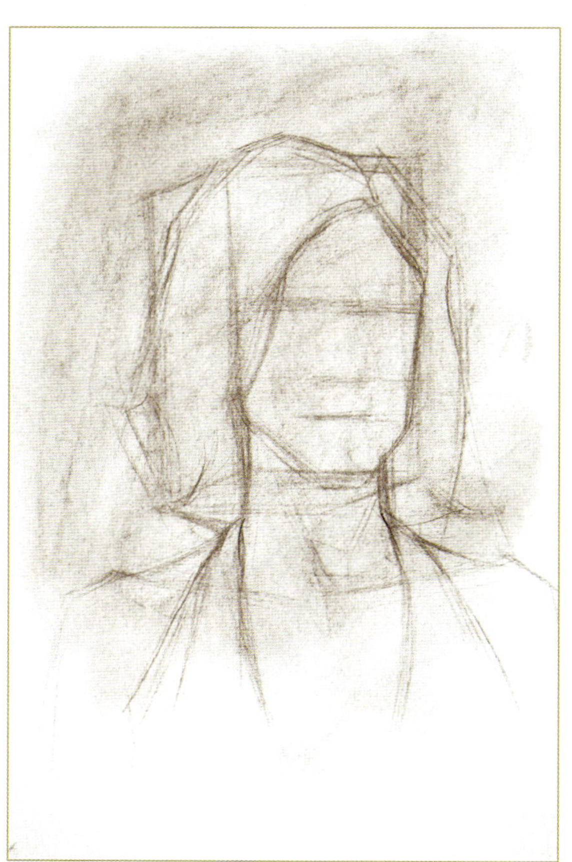

**3.** *Begin lightly constructing the contours of basic shapes, transforming the box of the head into a more human-looking relationship of masses. Add the neck and shoulders.*

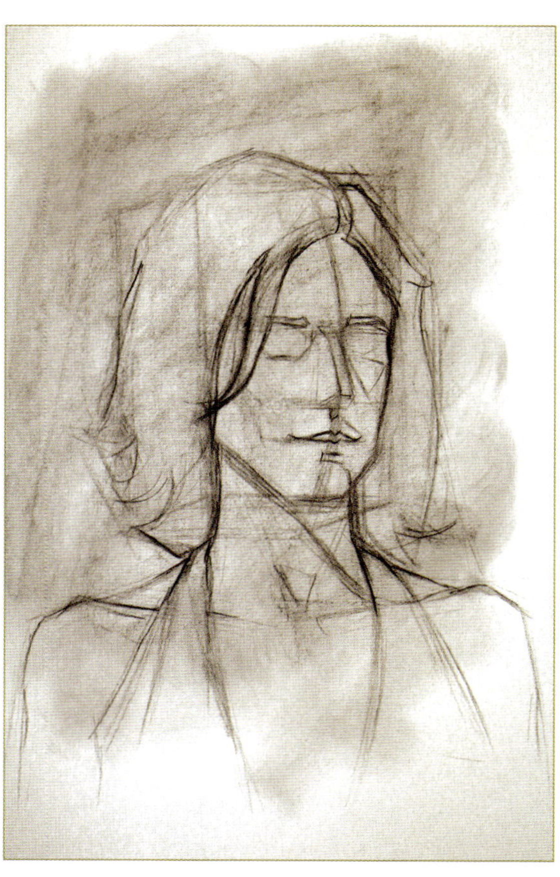

**4.** *Now switch to an HB charcoal pencil, which contains compressed charcoal and adheres more permanently to the paper. As you build the facial features, be sure to have a centerline reinforcing the direction in which the head is looking. Slowly become more specific with the masses, and remember to measure and check angles as you progress.*

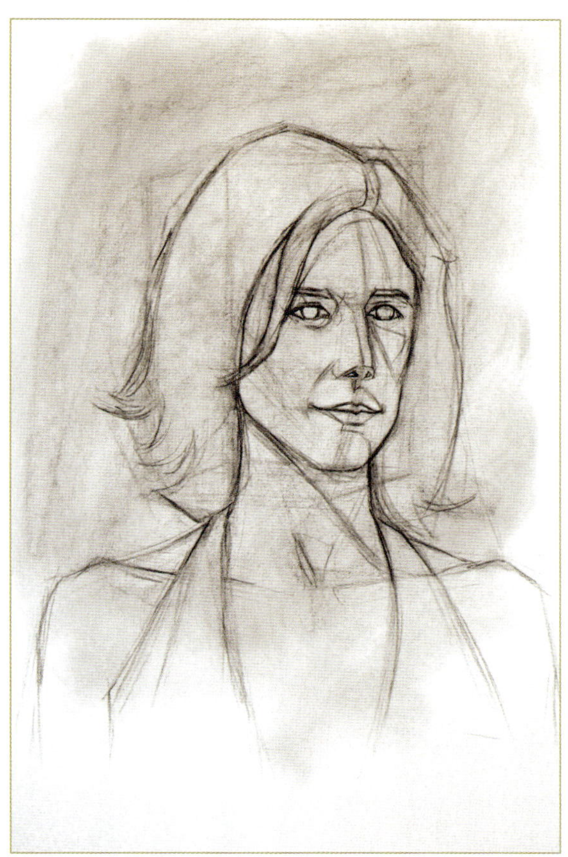

**5.** *Solidify your drawing and add details, capturing the way the light falls on the face. Use a darker line weight to bring out the focal points of the facial features.*

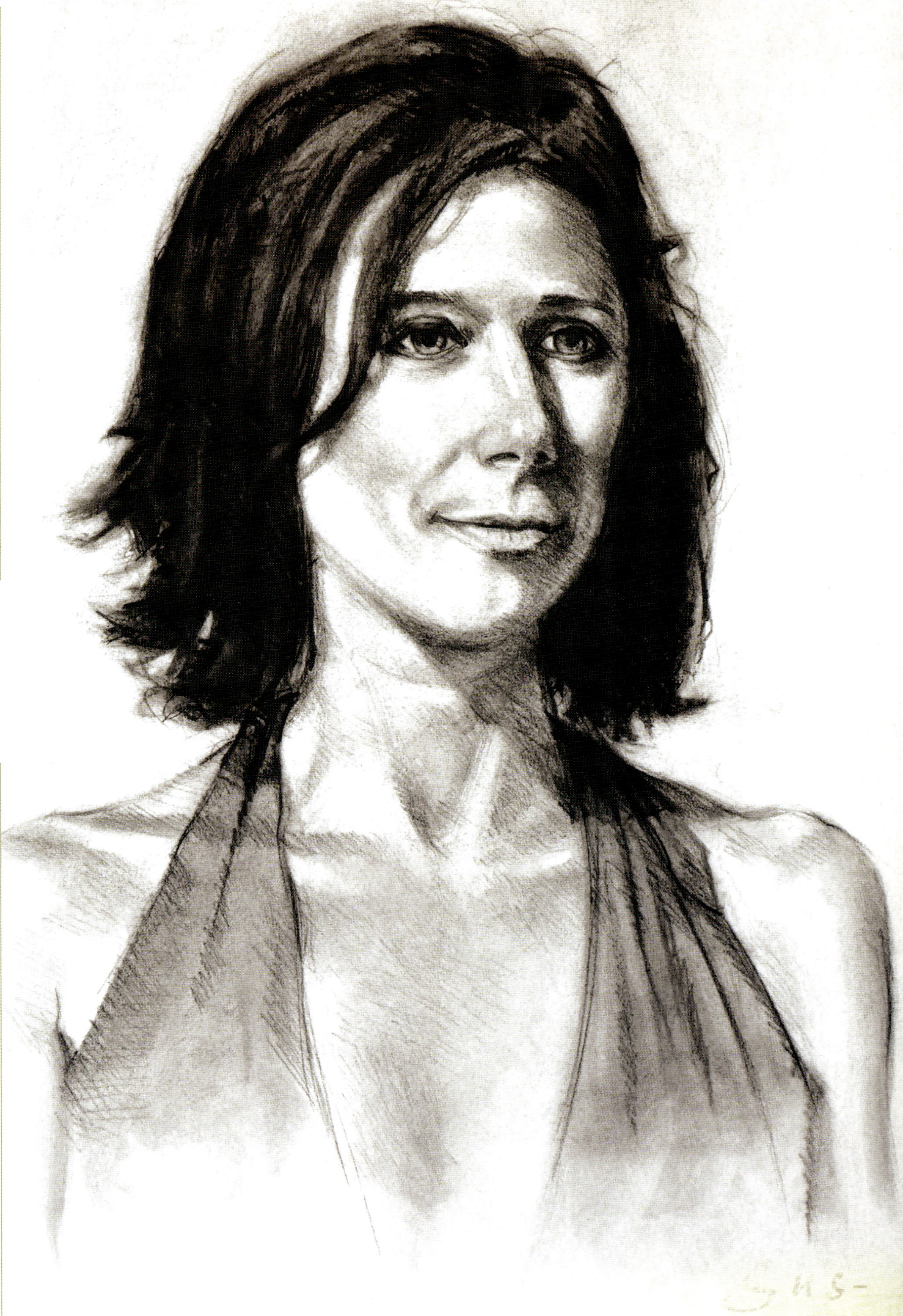

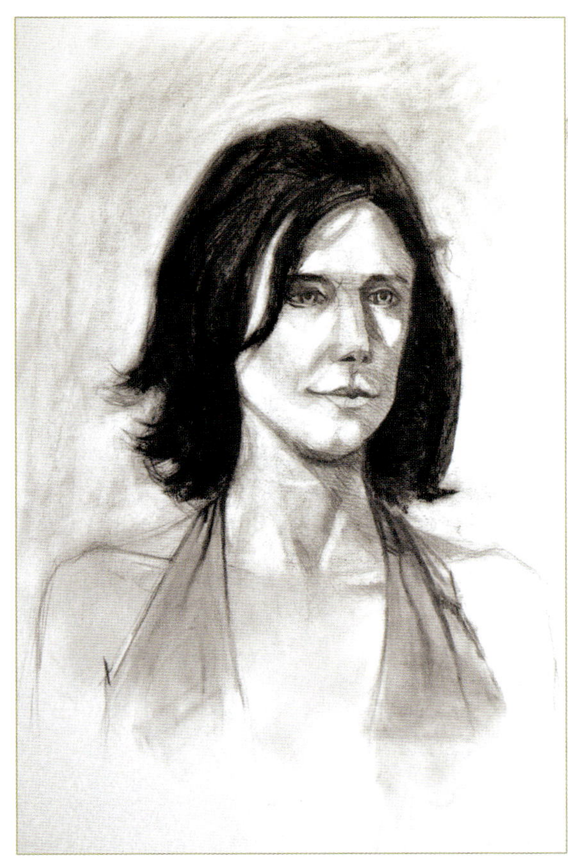

**6.** *With a stick of soft compressed charcoal, block in the dark hair, and lightly block in the clothing to reach proper local values; then smear with a chamois. Come back in with a soft charcoal pencil to darken what you've wiped away. With a kneaded eraser, begin separating the figure from the background and pull out highlights by removing the charcoal tone around the head and within the figure.*

**7.** *With both the kneaded eraser and electric eraser, remove the charcoal in areas that receive light in the figure to create subtle variation. Create soft and hard edges for your shadow shapes. Use your softer charcoal pencils to further push your darks. Back and forth, push and pull lights and darks using the erasers and pencils until the rendering is complete. Personally, I prefer a healthy combination of direct mark and smoother, wiped tone.*

# Black and White Media on Toned Paper

Using black and white media on toned paper is one of my favorite drawing techniques. This process, which usually involves middle gray toned paper, black charcoal, and white charcoal, can produce an amazing range of value that results in a breathtaking degree of realism. When done correctly, this technique is similar to the art of painting. Value is the first thing the eye sees—even before color and shape. Leonardo da Vinci was known for his ability to see and depict many variations of tonal gradients, yielding some of the world's greatest works of art.

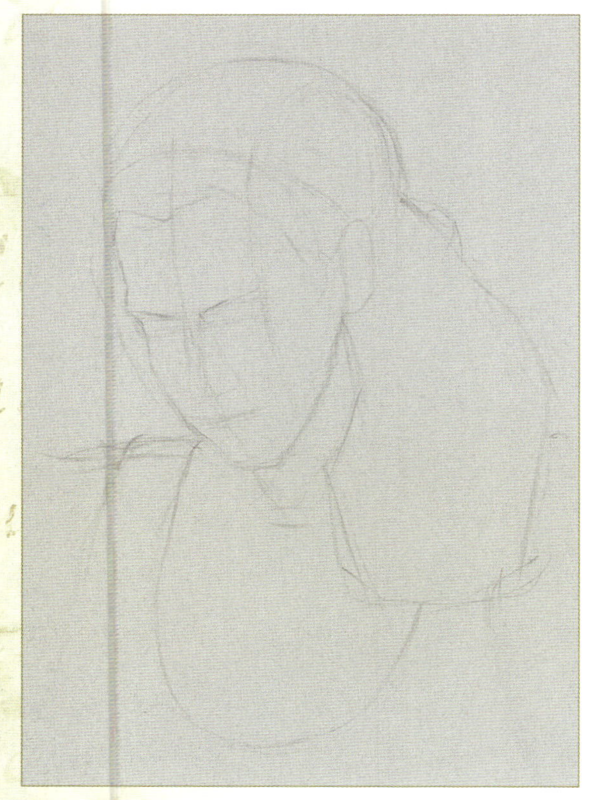

**1.** *Using vine charcoal, start your drawing on the smoothest side of the paper. Vine charcoal is easy to remove when mistakes are made. Construct the major planes of the face with a centerline showing the direction of the subject's gaze. Then indicate the basic masses and add measurement lines.*

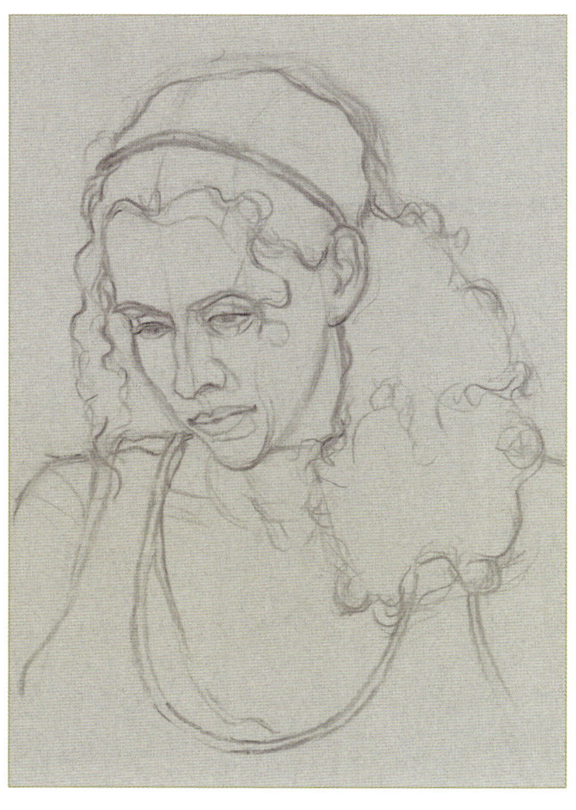

**2.** *Construct the drawing with light lines and separate value shapes. At this point, be more sensitive as you add the contour line, and begin communicating the different textures. Measure and check your angles, always starting with simple shapes first.*

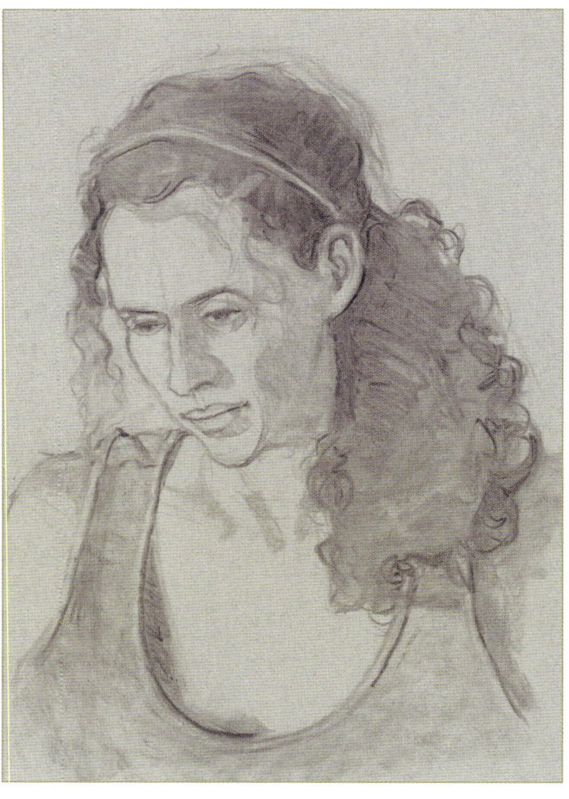

**3.** *The paper's value will be used as part of the value structure. Begin blocking in darker values with vine charcoal. Block in the hair with even tone, applying more charcoal for shadow shapes in large areas. Use broad strokes and turn the vine stick on its side, moving quickly.*

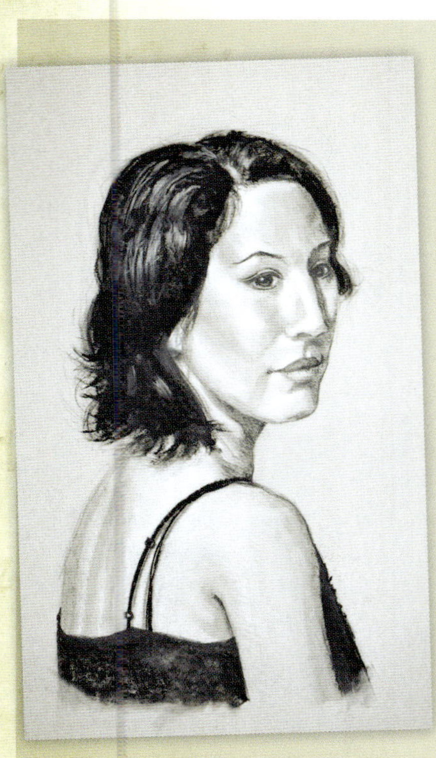

## Toned Paper

**Toned paper is available in a variety of values and colors. Some middle-tone grays are warm and some are cool. The gray drawing paper used in the piece at left is cooler and lighter than the paper used in the step-by-step project. Earth-toned paper is also a popular choice for this technique. Try several different papers to find the surface you like best.**

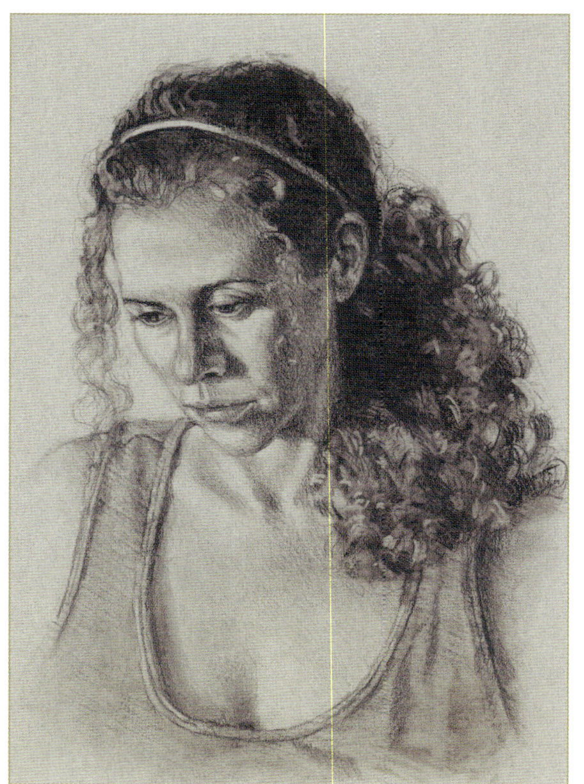

**4.** *Now use your charcoal pencils to render the entire piece. Use the B pencils for the darker areas and HB for the lighter tones. Smudge the charcoal to smooth out the tone. Within the hair, use the buildup of marks on top of the smudged tone to create textural differences. Use erasers to remove charcoal in unwanted areas and add highlights in the hair. Remember to incorporate variations in mark, value, and edge quality.*

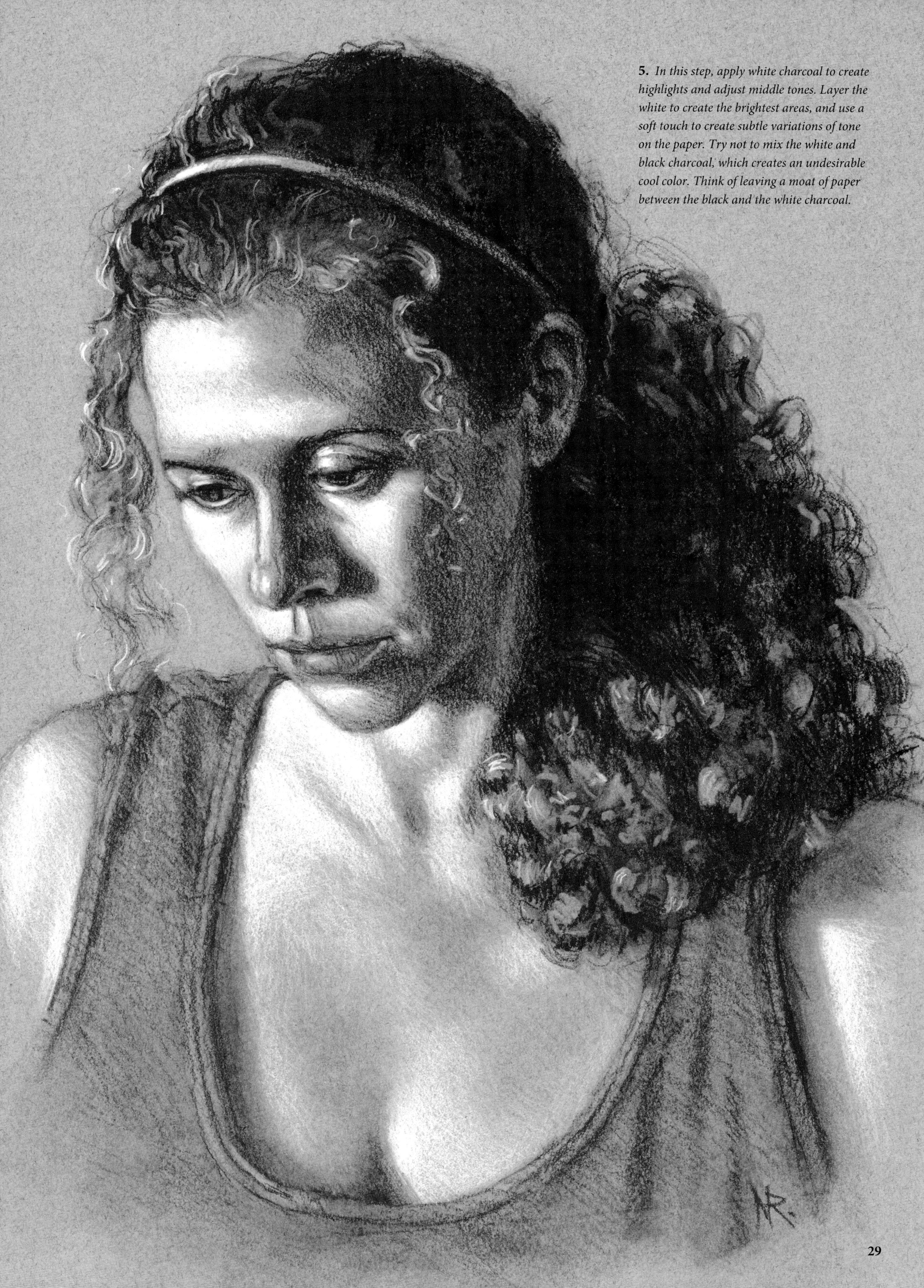

**5.** *In this step, apply white charcoal to create highlights and adjust middle tones. Layer the white to create the brightest areas, and use a soft touch to create subtle variations of tone on the paper. Try not to mix the white and black charcoal, which creates an undesirable cool color. Think of leaving a moat of paper between the black and the white charcoal.*

# Pastel Portrait

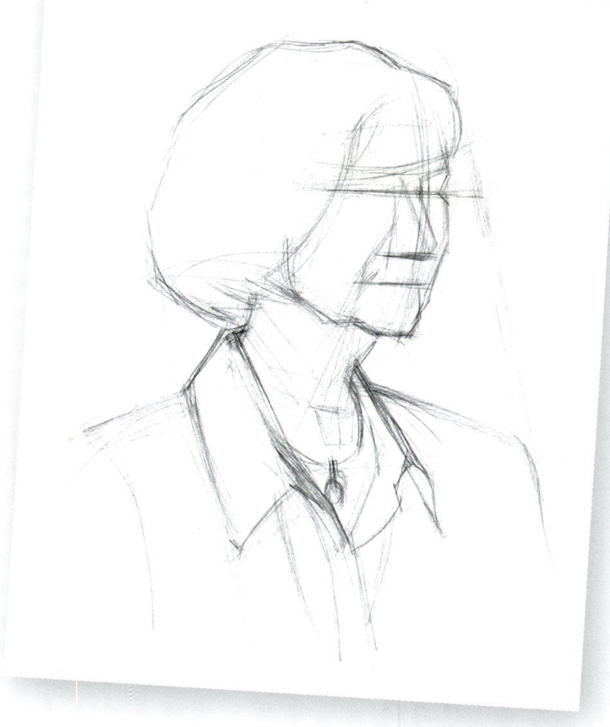

**Pastel offers a way** to develop your understanding of color while utilizing and developing fundamental drawing skills. This is as close to painting as you can get without using wet media. Start the drawing with graphite lines and then move to a monochromatic separation of light and dark with pastel, establishing the value structure before introducing more colors. When the pastel drawing is complete, you'll find that it has a warmth and vibrancy that is not achievable with graphite, pencil, or even toned paper and charcoal.

▶ **1.** *Create a line drawing in graphite on hot-press watercolor paper. Place the measurements for the eyes, nose, and mouth. Then construct the contours, checking your angles and using variation in line weight to lead the viewer's eye.*

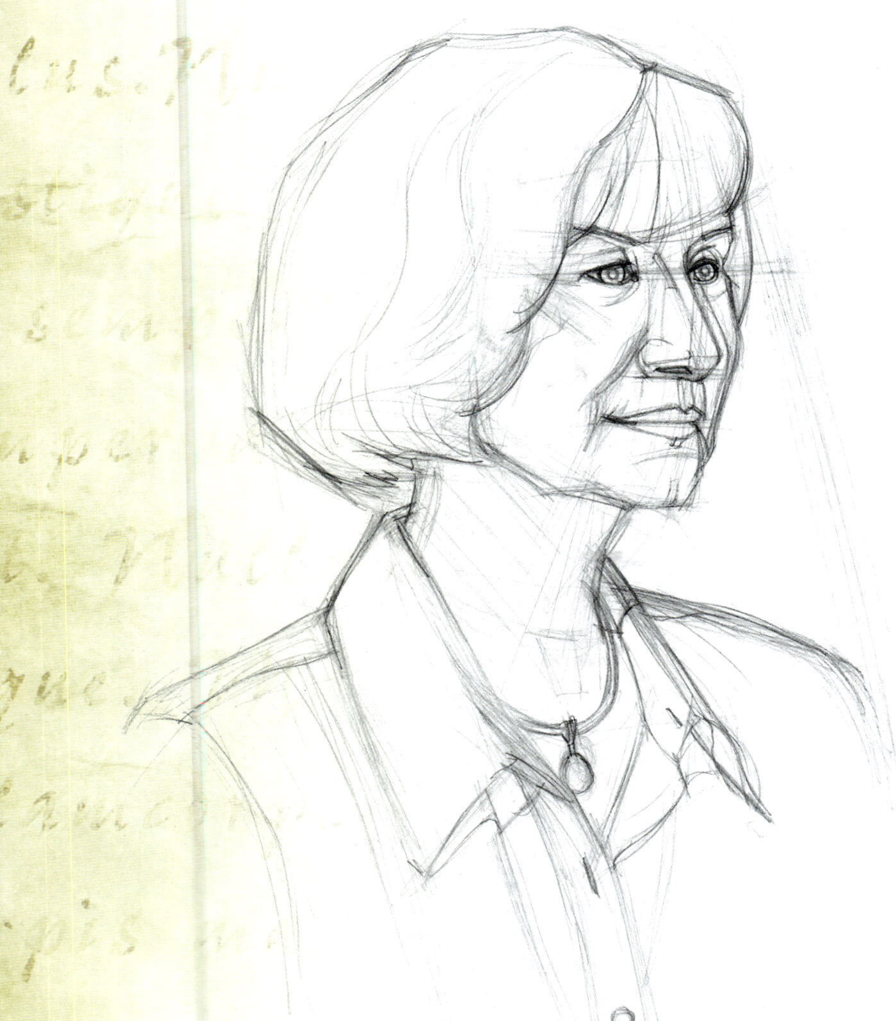

**2.** *Finalize the graphite drawing by closing all the shapes. Then develop the major and minor planes of the face, head, neck and shoulders. Create construction lines that show a logical variation of value or weight. Separate shadow shapes and reveal the subject's form using cross-contour marks.*

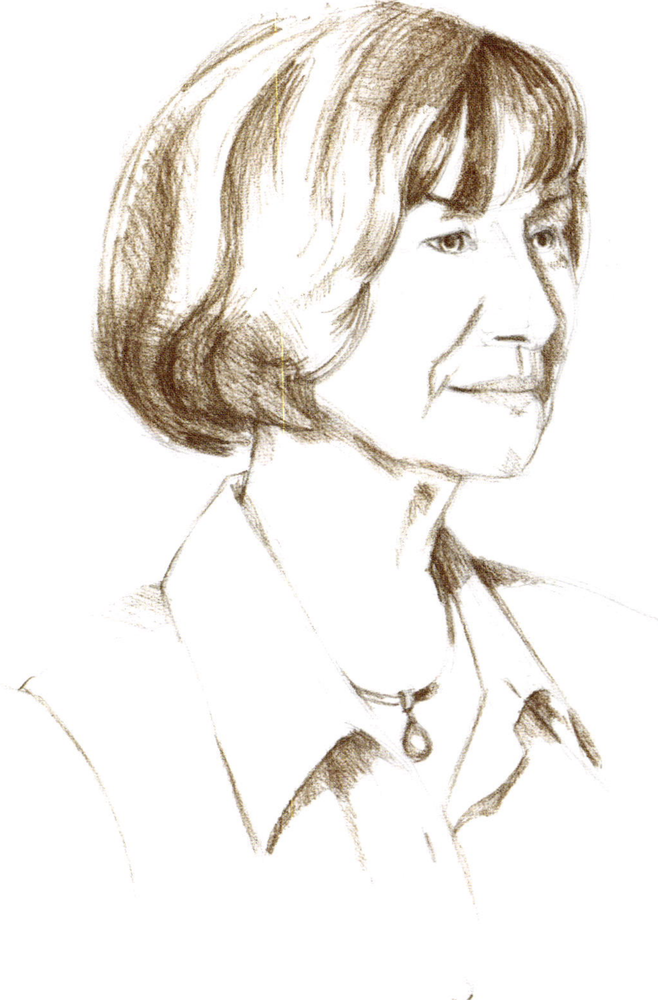

**3.** *Using a brown pastel pencil, establish the basic light logic and create the overall value structure. Squinting will help determine what comes first; start with the darkest darks and avoid focusing on detail at this point. Build up the whole drawing slowly and evenly.*

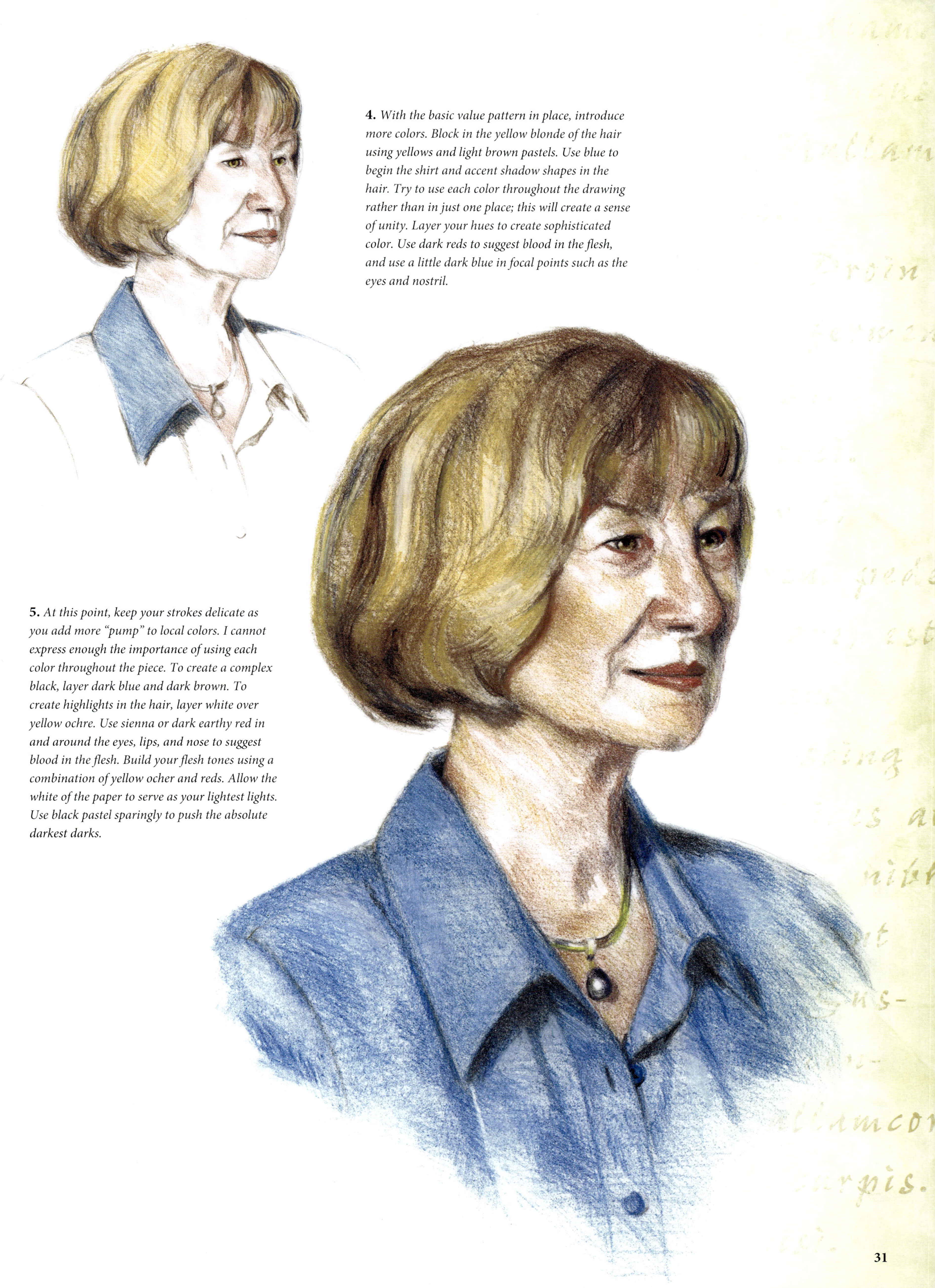

**4.** *With the basic value pattern in place, introduce more colors. Block in the yellow blonde of the hair using yellows and light brown pastels. Use blue to begin the shirt and accent shadow shapes in the hair. Try to use each color throughout the drawing rather than in just one place; this will create a sense of unity. Layer your hues to create sophisticated color. Use dark reds to suggest blood in the flesh, and use a little dark blue in focal points such as the eyes and nostril.*

**5.** *At this point, keep your strokes delicate as you add more "pump" to local colors. I cannot express enough the importance of using each color throughout the piece. To create a complex black, layer dark blue and dark brown. To create highlights in the hair, layer white over yellow ochre. Use sienna or dark earthy red in and around the eyes, lips, and nose to suggest blood in the flesh. Build your flesh tones using a combination of yellow ocher and reds. Allow the white of the paper to serve as your lightest lights. Use black pastel sparingly to push the absolute darkest darks.*

**Head drawing is challenging** and requires practice, patience, and time to master. I advise you to avoid relying on a particular formula to create your drawings; respond to each subject as an individual. Utilizing the techniques and exercises from this book will help you do just that. This art form can lead you on pathways, both to portraiture and to fine art. Both approaches to the head are timeless and serve different masters. Portraiture tests your skills at creating a likeness and an accurate representation of the subject. However, fine art is driven by personal expression; the translation of the subject is solely up to the artist and is based on a dialogue with art history.

With this book I intend to build and reinforce the foundation of head drawing for the beginner, as well as help the more advanced student gain further understanding. If you practice these skills through hundreds of drawings, I believe you will be on the path to success. As you practice, remember that drawing from life is imperative to an artist's success. There is nothing in art more rewarding than drawing the human form—it is absolutely the ultimate subject to master.

---

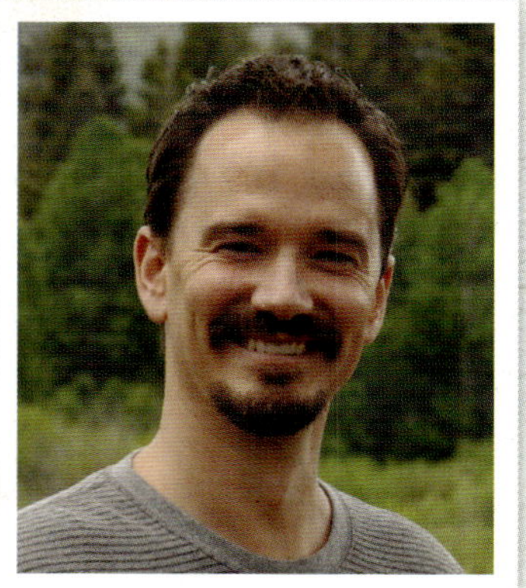

NATHAN ROHLANDER'S fine artwork is a contemporary approach to realism grounded in the figurative tradition. His artwork is sold in galleries both domestically and internationally. With an MFA in drawing and painting from California State University, Long Beach, and a BFA with honors in illustration from the Art Center College of Design, Rohlander currently teaches at several southern California colleges, including Laguna College of Art and Design.